FIGHTING
FOR
SURVIVAL

"Dr. Fitzroy Dawkins has done an extraordinary job of capturing and contextualizing the complex and contradictory relationship African Americans have with the practice of American medicine. He provides a path to better cancer outcomes for African Americans by pointing out that while it's important to remember your history, it's critical not to become a captive of it.

—Mike Jones, two-time cancer survivor,
award-winning columnist for the *St. Louis American*

"As an African American Clinical Pastoral Educator, I have been privileged to serve in major healthcare systems, providing spiritual care for patients, as well as educating students for healthcare chaplaincy. Through my years of ministry in this context, I am fully aware of the emotional roller coaster of fear, guilt, suffering, and denial that many patients experience. Dr. Dawkins has written a book that offers hope in the midst of despair. It's a book about overcoming the odds. It reveals a better future for African Americans through the promise of clinical trials. Read it! Discuss it! Be blessed by it!"

—Reverend Samuel Bryan,
ACPE Certified Educator Advent Health System

"The book our culture needed! A powerful and clear-eyed look at healthcare and clinical trial research in communities of color. An absolute must read! A pointed reminder of our obligation to not only remember the painful lessons of Tuskegee but to also actively participate in clinical research, ensuring that future breakthroughs include representation from minority communities."

—William Garrett, Sr., MBA,
SVP, Global Clinical Operations & Head,
US Business Operations at Ascentage Pharma

"Dr. Fitzroy Dawkins skillfully writes of the historical challenges people of color have endured when dealing with the healthcare system, while connecting the reader's attention to its present-day opportunities. I highly recommend this book."

—D'Brickashaw Ferguson,
NFL Alumni, Future Healthcare Professional

FIGHTING
FOR
SURVIVAL

CONQUERING CANCER AND THE AFRICAN AMERICAN PATIENT

FITZROY DAWKINS, MD

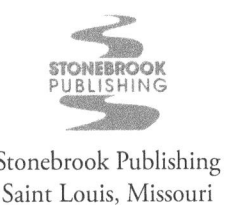

Stonebrook Publishing
Saint Louis, Missouri

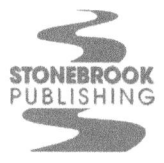

A STONEBROOK PUBLISHING BOOK
©2023, Fitzroy Dawkins, MD

This book was guided in development and
edited by Nancy L. Erickson, The Book Professor®
TheBookProfessor.com

Library of Congress Control Number: 2023918822

Print ISBN: 978-1-955711-33-3

www.stonebrookpublishing.net
PRINTED IN THE UNITED STATES OF AMERICA

This book is dedicated to my mother, Hazel Hyacinth Dawkins, the consummate British-trained nurse in the tradition of Florence Nightingale. Her love and steadfast support for me, her son, determined at all costs to be a doctor, has been a North Star for me. The examples she set as a health care practitioner, sometimes at significant risk to herself, have been a beacon that continues to light the way for me to be the best that I can be. At times, she is coaxing but always encouraging. I hope she is proud of the physician I have become.

Love,
Fitz

CONTENTS

INTRODUCTION

*"History and today's deplorable African American
health profile tell us clearly that black Americans need
both more research and more vigilance."*

—Harriet A. Washington, Medical Apartheid

The bitter vestige of winter disappeared, giving way to a beautiful and glorious spring day. That year, I attended the annual meeting of the American Society of Clinical Oncology (ASCO), held in beautiful Chicago, the Windy City. No street is quite like the Magnificent Mile with its splash of colorful flowers, skyscrapers, memorable restaurants, high-end shops, and the buzz and whirl of people rushing about. ASCO is the premier annual clinical science-driven cancer conference, and it's held in the United States. For many in the global oncology community, this is a must-attend cancer convention. It's a convergence of oncology nurses, oncology-focused physician assistants, award-winning oncology/hematology fellows, and the who's-who of prominent medical oncologists, clinical scientists, surgeons, and radiation oncologists. Biotech executives, drug sales representatives, as well as the FDA executives attend. ASCO conventions are geared toward education, cutting-edge advances in clinical oncology, and hematologic oncology research.

1

One of the highlights is learning about the critical results of clinical trials from across the United States and around the world. ASCO is an assembly for robust scientific and oncology-specific debates, discussions, and scientific disagreements. A place where new data challenge old dogmas, dogmas that sometimes die hard under withering science-based critique. Like a flash mob, twenty to thirty thousand persons descend upon Chicago for five days, and when business is concluded, they evaporate back to their home cities.

But meeting at ASCO serves another function. It's a forum and gathering of old acquaintances and colleagues who reestablish old bonds, talk shop, and share clinical practice war stories. This particular year was no different. I had prearranged to meet an old medical school colleague. We had gone our separate ways to different residency programs in different cities. But, quite unintentionally, we both followed our training in internal medicine with fellowships in hematology and medical oncology. We hadn't seen each other for more than five years. We discussed some of the highlights presented at ASCO that were of mutual interest and complained about the challenges we faced in our institutions and our research careers.

Then we chatted about our kids. He had a daughter, Annie, a gregarious life-of-the-party young woman, intelligent and accomplished. When she was in fifth grade, Annie's teacher suggested she had the aptitude to become a great attorney. As is often the case, a teacher can have an outsized positive impact on a child's life. The thought of becoming an attorney was a career guiding light for Annie as her high school years progressed.

My friend and his wife also agreed with the teacher's assessment and encouraged what appeared to be a sure-footed career trajectory for Annie. Her siblings were on board and teased her about what kind of lawyer she would be. Would she be "the people's lawyer," or would she be "a sell-out" and go for the money? Annie was accepted to the prestigious Duke University (Ivy League South) in Durham, NC, for her undergraduate work. Her path was set with a degree in the liberal arts, and then, she would be on to law school.

Somewhere during her undergraduate years, Annie had a change of plans. My friend heard echoes of doubt about her chosen path. Her dad dismissed any thought or mention of her striking out in a different direction. In his mind, that would never happen. The only way forward was for her to go to law school. There was no other option. Three years into her under-graduate work, thoughts of the LSATs, LSAT tutoring, the fuss, the flurry, and the stress associated with application to the best law schools set in. After graduating from Duke with a degree in hand, Annie came home with a different plan.

"Dad," Annie told her father while they were sitting at the kitchen table, "I'm not applying to law school."

"What do you mean 'I'm not applying'? You can't be serious."

Exasperated, he hauled his lanky frame up from a slumped posture. "But this is who you are," he said. "You've got the brains, the chops, the grades, and the assertiveness to be a top-notch legal scholar."

"Well," she said, "I'm sorry to disappoint you, but it's not going to happen. I've reconsidered."

As my friend described it, dismay and frustration within the family followed. She had been principally driven by her dad's ambition for her, and perhaps, he sought to live a bit vicariously through his daughter.

"I plan to get a job and then apply to business school," Annie explained.

Her first job, which she hated, was in Connecticut. But since her career trajectory was to get an MBA in a few years, she told herself the drudgery, low salary, and sweatshop men-tality of the company would be brief compared to the rest of her life. *They may take my body, but I will not give them my soul,* was her attitude. In between, there were multiple phone calls back home over the next two years.

With each call, as my friend ruefully drudged up from his memory, he asked—and perhaps even badgered Annie, "So, when will you sit for the LSATs? I will pay for an LSAT tutor if you need it," he reminded her. They would lock horns again and again. But Annie would not budge.

On one occasion, in sheer annoyance, she exclaimed, "Dad, I have no interest in law school, no desire to study law, and I'm tired of telling you. I need to find my way."

For the next few months, he didn't hear from Annie because she was frustrated. He, on the other hand, was confident that a career in law would be a financial winner. She didn't have to practice law if she chose not to. A law degree, he reasoned, would provide a robust platform for establishing a start-up.

Annie had realized that there were many attorney traps: the toxic relations junior partners have with their work, the many hours it takes to make partner, working all night and weekends too, the indignities suffered on the way to partnership, the sharkish nature of the business, and the lack of self-care that comes with the struggle of working in a law firm.

"Dad," she said, "some attorneys now describe themselves as 'recovering attorneys,' meaning the love affair with practicing law is over. There's a high burnout rate. I want no part of that."

Annie had taken a long, hard look. She'd done her homework on the legal profession; she understood the risks, the benefits, and the prestige associated (at least in theory) with the practice of law. Taken together, she didn't like what she saw. She saw another future—a better future—for herself and for the future family she hoped to have.

Annie's dad is of a different generation. His ambitions and advice for her were based on experience, history, and his understanding of a world that was consistent and predictable, tried and true. He was a physician with a good income, and he had Annie's best interest at heart. She, on the other hand, saw a future not so different from her dad's ambitions for her but one that required new approaches and a different way of thinking.

Annie's dad was old school. Annie knew that while prestigious, many law graduates were saddled with a mountain of debt and a poor quality of life post-graduation. Unless she attended a prestigious law school and graduated in the top 10 percent of the class, the promised wealth and high status could be elusive. She had surveyed the legal landscape and didn't accept her dad's viewpoint, even though it was well intended.

The Dangers of Groupthink

The Encyclopedia Britannica defines groupthink as a "mode of thinking in which individual members of small cohesive groups tend to accept a viewpoint or conclusion that represents a perceived group consensus, whether or not the group members believe it to be valid, correct, or optimal."

In her February 2020 essay, "Black Groupthink and Fused Identity: An Observation," Dr. Cynthia Alease Smith, a self-described anti-racism/anti-white supremacy essayist, said, "Black people are still in *a constant struggle of defiance* against that which sets itself up as superior and creates mechanisms, laws, regulations, rules, and behaviors to ensure the fallacy remains intact." (Emphasis mine.)

Reflecting on my conversation with Annie's dad in Chicago, I wondered if he, too, was a victim of a kind of groupthink. His recommendations were honed by years of observing the American professional landscape and mentally documenting what upward mobility and living the American dream looked like. Annie agreed with her dad's end goals. But she believed that a newer and better path was necessary.

Smith's article is a powerful reminder of how some Black American patients view the US medical care system, the historical inequality of care, and the advances made necessary through investigating new drugs in human beings, also known as *clinical trials*. Clinical trials are often seen as a "creation by the other." Created by the majority for the majority to serve themselves—the majority. Thus, the groupthink goes: *To participate—or, better yet, to succumb to—a clinical trial means that Blacks don't understand the long-standing "games" White people have played against "us." We must resist. We are being played for their financial and medical benefit. It may be suitable for "them," but it's not for "us."*

By extension, this prevailing attitude of mistrust and resistance extends to what some have called the *medical-industrial complex*. Here is how Arnold Relman, MD, described his version in a 1980 *New England Journal of Medicine* (NEJM) article: "The new medical-industrial complex is a large and growing network of private corporations engaged in the business of supplying health-care services to patients for a profit—services heretofore provided by nonprofit institutions or individual practitioners."

In the article, he makes it clear that he didn't include the pharmaceutical industry as part of that complex. But many patients today, both Blacks and Whites, beg to differ. They extend the definition to include today's biotech and pharmaceutical industries.

The reality is that there are centuries-old data on medical experimentation and exploitation of Black people in the United States. Harriet Washington, in her book *Medical Apartheid: The Dark History of Medical Experimentation in Black Americans from Colonial Times to the Present*, is steadfast in her documentation of the historical basis for this distrust. Thus, some Black Americans may argue: *The only way to ensure that we don't fall into the trap again is to maintain and perpetuate a posture of resistance. We should learn from our history, and a posture of mistrust is the best weapon we have against being misled again.* So, the narrative goes, *History tells us that no matter what we're told or by whom, or whatever the perceived benefit, we will be deceived. Just look at what happened in Tuskegee.*

So, the traditions—the groupthink—for a notable slice of Black Americans is to hold the line against the lies, especially when it comes to clinical trials. *They have hurt us in the past, and they will again. We have been fooled once, and we won't be conned again.* The fact that national apologies have been made, safeguards instituted against future abuse, and some Black American physicians and scientists have reached the highest echelons of the profession is of small comfort to some. That, by itself, is not enough to gain trust in the medical community.

> The reality is that there are centuries-old data on medical experimentation and exploitation of Black people in the United States.

There's a risk in persisting in this view, which has massive implications for the individual. No one wants to step out of the groupthink line. Many African Americans seem to say: *We have shared values and collective memories, and we will never allow bad things to be done to us as individual members of this collective. A good thing may pass us by, but how would we know if it's good for us? We'd rather wait to see the results of a clinical trial and then reap the benefits than run the risk of being a "guinea pig."*

The revolution in medicine is here and like a bullet train is hurtling down the track. The advances in managing patients diagnosed or at risk for cancer over the last fifty years have been breathtaking. Today, Black Americans can help shape their health narrative; the opportunity is unprecedented. Consider multiple myeloma, a type of bone cancer that impacts Black Americans at a much higher rate than Whites. Twenty percent of all new cases of multiple myeloma are diagnosed in Blacks. Scientists have some clues as to why that may be, but the answer is not very clear. We need the participation of Black patients to solve this riddle.

Another example is triple-negative breast cancer. For every White woman diagnosed with this condition, there are two Black women diagnosed with the same cancer. These are only two examples where Black Americans can help solve cancer puzzles that continue to defy clear answers.

> The revolution in medicine is here and like a bullet train is hurtling down the track. The advances in managing patients diagnosed or at risk for cancer over the last fifty years have been breathtaking.

Remember the high-flying Blackberry brand? At its peak in 2011, Blackberry had eighty-five million subscribers worldwide. It was an American icon that dominated the North American telecommunication landscape. When I joined pharma in 2005, I received my first Blackberry with great pride. I felt that I had "arrived," and, for me, owning a Blackberry was a symbol of my success as a biotech executive. President Obama had one, and it seemed the US Secret Service couldn't pry it from his side. It was a must-have for every business leader. Blackberries were so ubiquitous and conspicuous that they were lampooned as "the crackberry" because we were so addicted to them.

Then, Steve Jobs struck in 2006. When he introduced the first iPhone, he revolutionized the smartphone space. Almost overnight, the highly dependable Blackberry vanished; it crashed and burned as a business icon. Blackberry clung to the tried and true but never recovered their former glory. The Blackberry fell out of favor because the company didn't recognize (or ignored) the telecommunication revolution that was just over the horizon.

Why change when you have a good and consistent thing going, you ask? Because change is inevitable, and new problems require new methods and new solutions. Many Black Americans are stuck in the past, clinging to justifiable hurts and grievances. There's great wisdom in the West African saying known as Sankofa, a proverb of the Akan people. Translated, it says, "It isn't taboo to go back to the past and bring forward that which is useful." Sankofa symbolizes learning from experience, never forgetting the past, but leveraging the past to build a better future.

The vestige of slavery continues to rear its ugly head every day. It's most evident in our health care system

> **Many Black Americans are stuck in the past, clinging to justifiable hurts and grievances.**

with poor access to quality care and quality health insurance, socially underserved zip codes, and—for many African Americans—disrespect within the very health care systems that purport to be in their best interest. Fortunately, some large and prestigious academic centers in the United States, such as Rush Medical Center and Cook County Hospital, both in Chicago, acknowledge these historical facts and are committed to reversing some of the harm done. Harriet A. Washington, in her brilliant book of the same name, calls this medical apartheid. She goes on to observe, "History and today's deplorable African American health profile tells us clearly that black Americans need both more research and more vigilance."

Our past is stacked high with many triumphs and many positive lessons, and Black Americans can bring forward from our collective past that which is helpful, that which will lead us forward to more significant victories. In my experience as a Black medical oncologist, cancer is viewed in Black society as the implacable enemy, a boogeyman that's best ignored—which is a form of denial. And even when we find that the boogeyman is real, that cancer has invaded our very bodies, a transition from denial to hope takes place. But that hope is based on magical thinking. It's wishing and praying that cancer will go away but without a rational, scientific plan of attack. Praying is good and right, and hope is necessary, but it must be anchored to a logical, solution-oriented approach. I want our people to leverage, in the words of Malcolm X, "by any means necessary," the healthcare toolbox that's rightfully ours.

In my experience as a Black medical oncologist, cancer is viewed in Black society as the implacable enemy, a boogeyman that's best ignored—which is a form of denial.

Coupled with the dread of a cancer diagnosis is a fear or unwillingness to consider clinical trials as an option, even when the approved therapies can no longer strike down the Goliath we face. Yet, in other parts of society, African Americans have excelled as a people, striking back with great success against race-based misperceptions and slights. My sincere hope is that this book will shed some light on the advances being made in cancer therapy, inspire African Americans to be fearless in seizing the advanced cancer care opportunities available to all Americans, and embrace clinical trials as good medicine that can help secure their medical future and that of their children.

BUFFALO SOLDIER

"Fighting on arrival, fighting for survival."

—Bob Marley, "Buffalo Soldier"

"You're going to Buffalo for medical school? Do you know how cold it is? Do they even have any Black people there?" Shortly after saying things like, "Congratulations. You did it, Fitz!" and, "We always knew you could do it!" these questions came one after another from my family.

It was August in 1980s Buffalo, New York. Yes, *that* Buffalo—lush and green, pleasant and sunny. City lights, like a bejeweled diamond necklace, caress Lake Erie's night. Erie, so vast and expansive at first glance to the uninitiated, seemed to be the northern seacoast of the United States.

This was the Buffalo of my memories: home to waning Bethlehem Steel plants and Ford Assembly lines; proud supporters of the bluest of blue-collar sports, the Buffalo Sabers and Buffalo Bills; and the original Buffalo chicken wings, first introduced by the Anchor Bar. Oooh, those wings! Tangy and spicy with blue cheese, celery sticks, and shards of carrot. I can still taste them now. Delaware Avenue, "Millionaires Row," with its decades-old trees, impressive mansions, and high, leafy green hedges, at once enfolding the residents while simultaneously keep strangers at bay. The Avenue recalls a rich industrial past, home to captains of industry from a bygone era.

Buffalo is a bastion of medical advances. It's the birthplace of Dr. Sydney Farber, who years earlier made significant contributions to childhood leukemia, and Dr. Wilson Greatbatch of Greatbatch-heart pacemaker fame. Roswell Park Cancer Institute was another, a proud legacy of cutting-edge medical research, reported to be the oldest cancer center in the country.

This is where I landed—rather, where I exited the Amtrak train from New York City. It was August, but the winds swept over vast Lake Erie and warned of a chilly fall to come and an even more bitter winter. I was here to continue my trek to medical school, which began when I was a preteen in a land so very far away.

My first recollection of medicine and the calling it became for me was in Jamaica when I was six years old. My father piled my sister and me into a very typical and ubiquitous British automobile, the Austin.

"Where are we going, Daddy?" I asked.

"We are going to pick up your mother from the hospital in Montego Bay."

My mother was a nurse who worked the late shift at the old public hospital perched alongside a cliff overlooking the impossibly blue and green-tinged Caribbean Sea in downtown MoBay, as the locals affectionately called Montego Bay. We sat in the car while my older sister and I played games to entertain ourselves.

Finally, my mother emerged through the front door of the hospital. Among the many things she had with her was a large, closed container, which she handed to us in the back. It contained gauze and scissors. Our job (my sister's and mine) was to cut pieces of gauze from a long swaddle, fold these smaller pieces into dressings, and pile them neatly together in a separate container. My mother took these dressings back to the hospital the next day to use in her nursing duties. Much later, I learned that before these pieces could be used to dress wounds, they first had to be sterilized by a process called autoclaving.

This was Jamaica, my own Jamaica, measuring 146 miles long by fifty-one miles wide, a muscular little island at full stature of 4,411 square miles. As the locals say, "We may be little, but we tallawah," which means, "We may be small, but we are powerful." This island is a member of the British Commonwealth, nestling just ninety miles south of Castro's Cuba. This is where I thrived, filled with stories of Captain Morgan and the Pirates of Port Royal, runaway slaves known as the marrons who battled the English powers to achieve freedom and the right not to be enslaved—an island nation imbued with the love of politics, debate, and dominos. Here, I was disciplined and educated under an unforgiving British pedagogy, where ambition and competition were the life-giving blood that coursed through the island's arteries and veins. It was my home for the first eighteen years of my life, my home forever.

Post WWII, local islanders like my mother, who were the brightest and best of their generation, traveled by ship to the mother country, England, to be trained in various aspects of the healthcare professions. A distinct hospital odor of chloroform and carbolic soap was ushered into our car with my mother's arrival. It's a fragrance I remember to this day. Thus was my entry into the world of medicine as I understood it then.

My mother was the consummate professional nurse, trained in the rigors of the British nursing practices that emphasized discipline and duty no matter the cost. While in the United Kingdom, my mother was also trained as a midwife. Returning to Jamaica, she was hired by the national government. She was transferred many times to very rural parts of the country, where she was expected to be the nurse, the midwife, the doctor, and the dentist for the village. Why the doctor and the dentist? Because these professionals were as rare as a hen's tooth. The villagers were lucky if the doctor came to the village more than once per month. The dentist was even more sporadic. My mother was the medical professional who was able to manage until such time. On occasions, "Nurse," as she was affectionately called, was summoned by a young boy sent by his parents because the "baby soon come," meaning his mother was about to deliver. The journey into the bush took her over rough and hilly terrain often inaccessible by car, where traveling even short distances could take an hour. Many times, the baby did not come right away, and because there were no hospitals for miles around, she would sometimes stay for days until there was actual labor and a baby was finally delivered.

These were my formative years. I had no idea at that time the indelible impact her example would have on me as a young oncologist many years later. My final stop in my formal Jamaican education was at Wolmer's Boys (High) School, a prestigious and highly sought-after public institution founded in 1729. Our inspiring motto was *Age Quod Agis,* which is Latin for *Whatever you do, do it well.*

I'd had significant career discussions with my mother about my next steps, about achieving my dreams, and how to accomplish them. In her view, I needed to make a change. She thought I needed to leave behind the only country I'd ever known. I had to leave my comfort zone—my country, my friends, the island beaches, and a sense of belonging. I left with a heavy heart and a single-minded purpose to become a physician and to return to my island in the sun. The memory of the shortages of doctors in my native land made a deep impression on my teenage mind.

As I embarked on my American odyssey, I reflected on one of the driving forces that led me to the monumental decision to pursue a career in medicine. While living in rural Jamaica, when I was ten or eleven years old, I became very ill with severe right hip pain, a high fever, and listlessness. This was very uncharacteristic for a boy who enjoyed the outdoors and playing cowboys and Indians and marbles with his friends. The local doctors in the provincial parish capital of Mandeville weren't able to help. When all else failed, I was taken to UC, the University College of the West Indies, located in Mona, just north of the sprawling capital city of Kingston. They offered the highest standard of care. It was the training and proving ground for English-speaking Caribbean health professionals.

After my mom traveled to England in the 1950s, higher education institutions began to flourish in Jamaica, and the pressure to travel to England, Canada, or the United States diminished. The best physicians, surgeons, and allied health professionals practiced at UC. If no other institution on the island could figure something out, they would. And if they couldn't, the next stop was the United States or the UK. However, those options weren't available to me at the time. After a long wait in the emergency department, also known as Casualty, I was admitted.

Multiple tests and X-rays later provided a diagnosis, but since I was a child, I wasn't privy to what "it" was. Decades later, I tried to get information from my medical records but was unsuccessful. Neither was I able to reach some of the consummate professionals who took care of me. My best guess is that I had an infection of my right hip bone, known as Osteomyelitis. The course of care kept me in the hospital for months on end.

I had multiple surgeries on my right hip and wound drainage tubes, and I presume now, a course of antibiotics.

What I hated the most was the almost full-body cast made of Plaster of Paris. It extended from mid-chest down my right thigh and leg. I could only lay down and stand up. I couldn't sit because I was effectively straight-jacketed. Inside this hard cast, cotton had been wrapped around my body. The itching at times was unbearable, mainly because I couldn't reach some areas to relieve this sensory discomfort. In addition, my right leg was in traction for considerable periods. I was shuttled between the premier hospital at UC and a provincial hospital in Morant Bay, St. Thomas, which was necessary to ease the bed shortage at the premier UC. Finally, after five months of pain, itching, missed school, and longing to play as any young boy would, I was discharged and free from the dreadful cast and able to walk again.

The care I received from a consummate cadre of physicians, nurses, physical therapists, and a social worker was most memorable for me. But among them, two people stood out and probably sealed my ambitions to become a physician. The first was Professor John Golding, an English orthopedic surgeon, who had seen action in WWII and was inordinately kind to me and my plight as a sick schoolboy. The other, Dr. Rowe, was Professor Goldings's resident in training. Night after night, when he was on call, he'd come to see me when a nurse summoned him. Both were professional, thoughtful, and considerate and left a lifelong impression on me.

My mother knew I wanted to be a physician. In fact, my whole family knew; it was an inside joke. With high school completed, my mother decided that I should go to the States to pursue my ambitions. The debates between us—me making the case that I should not leave the island, I should not go to New York—were memorable, at least to me. Much to my chagrin, I lost that one.

This was a journey of firsts for me. I'd never been on a plane before; it was my first time leaving paradise, and I was ill-prepared for temperatures below seventy-five degrees. I landed at Kennedy Airport, Queens, New York, on a chilly April night, cold and shivering, with no one to greet me, accompanied only by a heart filled with dreams and ambitions. Upon arrival in a strange and very foreign land, I realized that I had to fight for survival. I was all I had, humanly speaking. People were coming and going, hugging hellos, waving goodbyes, or standing in line to wait for a taxi that pulled up in a long and endless yellow line. The sights, sounds, and odors were unfamiliar yet mesmerizing.

This should have been an exciting time for me, footloose and fancy-free. I was a teenager in New York City. But that wasn't the case. As an avid consumer of American television news and movies, the violent scenes I'd witnessed left me with a sense of foreboding. I stepped out into the cold spring night and went to the taxi stand. I fisted a handwritten note with a Queens, New York, address as if it were life itself. I showed the address to the driver, and I was off to Cambria Heights, just northeast of all places—Jamaica, Queens!

On arriving at my destination, I was greeted by my host family. The woman was a Jamaican nurse like my mother. They had met at Beth Israel Hospital in Manhattan when my mother had migrated to America before her return to Jamaica. They had a college-age daughter who also aspired to be a physician. My mother had arranged for me to live with my host family as a renter while I plotted my course toward medical school. In retrospect, I'd already embraced a line from Bob Marley's—a fellow Jamaican's—song, "Buffalo Soldier," released some years after my arrival: "Fighting on arrival, fighting for survival."

I was in an unfamiliar country with strange surroundings, customs, and systems. I needed to sort through how to support myself and apply to college. There were so many options. Which was best for me, and how would I finance my education?

I had a lot going for me, like an excellent command of English, a rigorous high school education, an exceptionally nurturing Jamaican expat family, and a West Indian-centric church group. Despite our frequent dustups about going to the US, in hindsight, my mother was brilliant! My host family's daughter was living at home, and she had already navigated the college application process. In fact, at the time, she was a sophomore. It was such a strange word—sophomore—to me. What better way to get advice about college, the choice of a major, tuition needs, and the social scene?

I felt intense pressure to succeed. After all, America is the land of opportunity. How could I go to America and "not make something of yourself"? This is what I imagined I'd hear from my fellow Jamaicans back home if I failed. I was driven to succeed; I needed to scale that mountain and silence the voices in my head.

But first things first. I had to find gainful employment to pay for my room and board. My mother made it clear that I had to find my way. To do that, I worked many temporary jobs. I unloaded trucks in the Garment District of Manhattan, waited on and served food to employees of the old JC Penny headquarters on Sixth Avenue, and worked the graveyard shift in a factory in the South Bronx of *Fort Apache, The Bronx* movie fame.

Coming to America was like landing in the center of an array of books, ideas, food, sports, and culture, all wrapped in one. And here I was in the heart of the Big Apple, the uniquely iconic New York City. I ate pizza for the first time, enjoying the Sicilian style most. In fact, a slice of Sicilian and a Coke at the local pizza joint near my college in Jamaica, Queens, was a lunch staple for me. I drank root beer for the first time and consumed large volumes of White Castle hamburgers. In short order, I became a New York Islanders hockey fan during their championship years. I discovered a few books by Black American authors, such as *Man-Child in the Promised Land* by Claude Brown and *The Autobiography of Malcolm X*, as told to Alex Haley, to name a few. I devoured them. I wanted to understand the culture. I wanted to absorb all the good things and understand some of the dark sides of America.

I enrolled in City University of New York's (CUNY) York College. My high school diploma was solid and could have afforded me entrance to a more prestigious college. But there was a practical reason for my choice. I had secured work at the M&T Bank located on Hillside Avenue in Queens. This meant I could ride my bike from home to college and to work and back home again, a tremendous cost-saving strategy.

I majored in biology. That made sense to me because it seemed to me, everyone who was pre-med majored in biology or chemistry. Only with the blessing of hindsight and ignorance of the system did I later realize that I could have enrolled in any major as long as the prerequisite pre-med coursework was met.

With a bachelor's degree in biology from City University of New York firmly in hand, I was accepted as a first-year medical student to State University of New York- Buffalo School of Medicine, the future Jacobs School of Medicine and Biologic Science. There were only ten Blacks in a class of almost 150 students. Those four years were the most academically rigorous that I and most of my classmates had ever faced. In our group of eight for Gross Anatomy—and, oh, the stench of it all—we labored together to dissect "Quincy," our cadaver named for a popular medical forensic TV show of the same name. Quincy was not young. He was balding. His skin was wrinkled, and it was clear from his internal sutures, surgical staples, and well-healed scars that he'd been acquainted with real doctors before he was assigned to us wannabees. The stench aside, it was fun, and all of us felt that, at last, we were on the path to becoming great Doctor of Medicine, at least in our minds.

Four years and a bevy of automobiles later, I graduated. My first beauty was a very early model, canary-yellow, stick-shifting Audi. It frequently stalled out, and transmission and oil leak issues abounded. One frosty morning, I chugged into a mechanic's shop after another oil leak and said, "It seems the car is leaking again. Could you check it out for me?"

Thirty minutes later, he said, "I wouldn't put another penny into this car. It is a piece of junk."

That isn't what I wanted to hear. So, I responded, "Thank you, but I would appreciate it if you could fix the problem. I need this car."

It turned out he was right. On another soul-freezing cold day, I was driving to classes at Millard Filmore Hospital. I came to a stop and waited for the light to change. I got the green light, but the Audi wouldn't—couldn't—move an inch. It died due to another overheated engine. The cause? Yet another oil leak.

Next came a charming Oldsmobile Cutlass Supreme of the very, very early model I was accustomed to. Two years after my Olds, four years after emerging from the Amtrack train in Buffalo, multiple apartments in questionable neighborhoods, two Asian roommates, and finally having my place neatly tucked under the stairway of an old colonial house from the Victorian era, like the troll in "Three Billy Goats Gruff," I reached my journey's end and earned my medical degree.

Along the way, I had some stark reminders that despite everything I'd done and worked so hard for, I was still seen as "the other" in this primarily blue-collar town dominated by second and third-generation residents from southern, eastern, and western Europe. When I was driving the yellow Audi, I'd moved into one of several antagonistic neighborhoods in

Buffalo. I woke up one morning to see that my canary-yellow car had been used as a canvas to express hatred. Parked in an alleyway and next to a police officer's home, the word *nigger* was written across my car in black scripted letters.

Seared into my memory forever was when I was confronted in the pre-dawn hours by four white men with Confederate flags flapping in the wind. My preferred place to study was in the basement of the medical school with a bucket of wings and a helping of carrot and celery sticks in tow. Around 1:00 or 2:00 a.m., I usually headed home, less than a half mile away. On my way home, I was forced to an abrupt stop. Four young men appeared to be on the hunt for prey, and it seemed I fit the bill. They stepped out of their car. They had one question, and I, alone at the time and fearing for my life, thought I only had one prayer left.

Their one question was, "Do you know how to spell .22 caliber?"

I froze. I did not—could not—speak. But I could pray, and that I did. There was, in fact, a ".22-caliber killer" (the notorious Joseph Christopher) who roamed Buffalo and was murdering Black men and boys. His reign of terror started before I arrived in the city and continued while I was there. After about two minutes—what seemed to me like an eternity—all four men returned to their car and sped away. My prayers were answered, and *Maybe, just maybe,* I thought, *I'll live to walk at my graduation.*

In the end, graduation was less a celebration and more of a relief. My long-envisioned dream had been achieved.

Hospital Training

Buffalo winters are legendary, and the howling winds off Lake Erie are like marauding Huns that cut through winter-armored clothes. Snowdrifts piled so high at times that they obscured lower-level house windows. I remember a particularly bone-crushing day in January when a snow emergency was declared, and the mayor banned all cars from the streets. Only emergency personnel were allowed. I was one of them.

"Fitzroy, can you get to the hospital this morning?" came the stern question from a hospital administrator.

"I'll try, but I'm not sure how. I live on Richmond Avenue, and as you know, because of the snowdrifts and all, it's too far to walk," I said. "Plus, my car is unreliable under the best of circumstances."

"Well," the administrator said, "You *are* essential personnel, and you're expected to report in. We'll send one of Buffalo's Finest to take you to ECMC. After your shift, your ride home is guaranteed."

"Thank you," I said. "I'll be there." I also thought, *Oh great, another first for me. The police showing up at a Black man's address. What will the neighbors think?* But duty called, and I was whisked away.

One morning, after an overnight shift, it was my turn to present at Morning Report. The night before had been jam-packed with admissions to the ICU, CCU, spinal taps, and blood smears to review. My two-by-four cards contained all the possible information my professor could ask or need to know about each patient who was admitted. I walked into the room. Just ahead of me was this stunning African American woman, also in a white coat, though shorter than mine. She wore a nicely pleated skirt and a red top. I stopped in my tracks. *I don't remember seeing her before,* I thought.

All at once, a silent conversation assaulted my brain: *How do I maneuver to ensure a meeting with her this morning? Who is she? Why is she in Morning Report, and how did I not see her before now?* The Morning Report was a blur. Afterward, I was determined to get answers and to get them from her.

She was a PharmD candidate at the SUNY School of Pharmacy on her clinical rotation at the flagship hospital, Erie County Medical Center. Having established base credentials and getting her telephone number, I quickly moved toward a possible date. Her answer was no. Sometime later, confident in my persuasive skills, I asked again. Her answer was less emphatic, but it was still, "No."

"But," she said, "Maybe at a different time when my course load is lighter."

Wounded and a little ticked off that she turned down a date with a *doctor,* I decided not to ask again. After much water under the bridge, we did have a first date and were married eighteen months later in my final year of training. The lights along the shores of Lake Erie never shone brighter.

In my eighth and final year in Buffalo, I worked as an internist for a prominent Black cardiologist in Buffalo, Dr. Kenny Gales. I took care of his patients with general internal medicine issues. With few exceptions, all were African American. In turn, this freed him up to focus on his large pool of cardiology patients. It was wonderful to work alongside an experienced and respected physician. It enriched, expanded, and deepened my skills as an internist. Because most patients were African Americans, caring for them on a weekly basis gave me an even greater appreciation of their struggles with the medical system. By night, I moonlighted in the ER and was contracted to work in emergency rooms across the region.

My wife received her doctorate and was appointed assistant professor at Howard University's School of Pharmacy in Washington, DC. At the same time, I began a three-year stint as a hematology/

> **Because most patients were African Americans, caring for them on a weekly basis gave me an even greater appreciation of their struggles with the medical system.**

oncology fellow at George Washington University Medical Center (GW), located in the Foggy Bottom area of our nation's capital. I was fortunate that a position was available for a first-year fellow because that meant my wife and I wouldn't have to suffer through a long-distance marriage, which can sometimes happen when you're still in medical training.

In my dual training in hematology and medical oncology, I was more interested in hematology. I looked in the microscope and enjoyed how a specimen would come alive after it was stained with the appropriate reagents. Bacterial cells, previously invisible to the naked eye, were like a miracle when visible through the microscope's lens. I could discern the concentration, the species of bacteria, etc. And a drop of blood on a glass slide, correctly stained, *Wow, what stories these slides could tell!* Cells came alive: red blood cells, red cells that were sickled, iron deficient red blood cells, white blood cells, leukemic cells, platelets that were distorted, big ones and small. Oh, the beautiful things I could see and the diagnoses I could make. Like needles in a haystack, the darkness could be illuminated under the glaring light of this ancient but still incredible, useful medical instrument. So, I started my fellowship skewed toward hematology, with no plans to change my career trajectory. But there was a pivotal moment. When or exactly how I'm not sure, but it was clear that my subconscious had quietly surveilled the medical world around me, and the pivotal moment was a total of all I had seen.

At first, medical oncology seemed so morbid, so painfully sad, so incredibly hopeless that I couldn't envision it as a career. But I'd developed a respect for my oncology-focused professors and how they approached their craft, the passion with which they debated and argued about the best course of care for each patient, their strong emphasis on research: bench research in a laboratory with Petri dishes and laboratory animals and clinical research focused on clinical trials. Each had a focus on advancing science, oncology treatment, and the lives of patients. Basic science shaped and informed clinical research. Clinical research based on treatment outcomes and cancer disease resistance drove the clinician back to the lab seeking new answers, then back again to clinical trials that could exceed the milestones previously achieved. They convinced me that the status quo in cancer care was not acceptable. To immerse myself in research was cancer patient care and advocacy of the highest order. I began to see patients in a more positive light and knew that effective treatment was possible and that some patients might even be cured. For me, clinical research opened many possibilities. It was a window for hope and the possibility of joy. I began to believe I could make a difference.

Seventeen years almost to the month after landing at JFK on that dark, chilly April Sunday, my formal training came to an end. Now, I had to decide on my career path. Would it be teaching or private practice? As I pondered

> I began to see patients in a more positive light and knew that effective treatment was possible and that some patients might even be cured.

my next move, I replayed the video of my life in my mind. I remembered the rejection I felt at the end of medical school, flush with a degree from a prestigious school, ready to execute a promise I made to return to my home country to give back. After my residency, I planned to return to Jamaica to teach and practice at UC, which had been pivotal in my early years. I wanted to help train the next generation of physicians. So, before my training was complete, I met with the chair of medicine at that time and told him as much.

He said in effect, "My dear Fitzroy, isn't it noble of you to want to return and help your fellow countrymen? Feel free to contact me again when your training is over."

But he gave me no sense of a warm welcome. No welcome for a native son. After that conversation, I felt somewhat presumptuous that I could have something to offer. I had no connection to the university's elite. With no clear explanation for the rejection I felt, I was left to wonder: *Would things have been different had I trained under the more familiar and, at the time, more respected British medical system?*

After that experience, I met with a Jamaican internist and cardiologist who had a private practice in Kingston, the capital city. Trained at Howard University as an internist, followed by a cardiology fellowship at a prestigious hospital in Boston, he'd returned home. He told me a similar story. He had returned to Jamaica, eager to teach and give his services. He, too, felt shunned by the establishment, so he started a private practice. He said it took him more than a decade before he, also a native, was accepted as one of their own. He was finally able to help in the teaching program at UC. Despite these difficulties, he encouraged me to come back home.

Years later, after multiple conversations with my Jamaican and African American families, with some bitterness, I accepted that a return to that jewel in the Caribbean was not optimal. To paraphrase Harry Belafonte, the famous calypso singer, "I was sad to say I would not be back for many a day."

Had I abandoned my dream? Was I in dereliction of duty—the same duty I witnessed in my mother, Dr. John Golding, and Dr. Rowe? The question still haunts me. But it also struck me that this great country of the United States of America had also given me much. More to the point, Black Americans, like my wife's family, who are from Virginia and North Carolina, have given me much. They've been in America for centuries. They had suffered greatly. In the 1960s, segregated Washington, DC, was still a reality. It was in this world that my wife was born. As she told the story, even in 1960s Washington, DC, pregnant Black women did not find the George Washington University Hospital a welcoming place to give birth.

Black people had lived through slavery and Jim Crow, and they had marched, fought, and died for their freedoms because they understood that they, too, were Americans with the same unalienable rights. When I arrived some years later, believing that I could apply to any medical school and expect to be admitted, it was because I stood on the shoulders of giants. The groundwork had already been laid. I owed the men and women a debt of gratitude. If Jamaica was no longer a possibility, how should I redirect my priorities?

Toward the end of my fellowship, my options were to go into private practice or an academic career. Private practice was predictable. I'd had a taste of it, and as vital as it was, I opted for an academic path. I felt at my best when I was probing, challenging, asking new questions, and seeking new solutions. After multiple rounds of interviews for a faculty position at either the University of Maryland's Greenebaum Cancer Center in Baltimore or Howard University College of Medicine, I received an offer from each, and I accepted the post at Howard.

Howard University

It was a heady time that was filled with endless possibilities. Here was my opportunity to give back. I was an assistant professor of medicine at a historically Black college and university (HBCU). I had an opportunity to practice, teach, and conduct clinical research and to follow in the footsteps of my mentors in a hospital whose original name was Freedman's Hospital. I met and worked with some of the best clinicians in their respective fields.

I also cared for some of the who's-who of prominent Blacks: a member of Congress, diplomates from West Africa and the Caribbean, physicians, and physicians' wives. I delivered medical care to the uninsured and the insured alike.

I was an assistant professor of medicine at a historically Black college and university (HBCU).

Here, I met patients from every walk of life who saw Howard University as their shining light on a hill, their beacon of hope from the harsh realities of care in other institutions. Howard University Hospital was a trusted institution.

High on my list of patients was a man from the South who was diagnosed with stage four colorectal cancer. One day, while on rounds with my team, I went to his room for a routine evaluation. In the process, I observed something I hadn't seen during my first contact with him. It was a keloidal scar, an irregular gash on one of his calves. I asked him a question, addressing him as "mister" as a sign of respect, so crucial in the African American community.

"Mr. Bridges, I'm sorry I missed this scar on your leg when I first examined you, but what happened here? This doesn't look like a surgical scar. Is it related to cancer surgery?"

I had a team of students, residents, and fellows with me, and I hoped to make an impression on them.

He responded, "Dr. Dawkins, no doctor has asked me that recently. Thank you. You know what happened at Selma, right?"

I nodded as I recalled the grainy black and white TV images of Dr. Martin Luther King and others marching over the Pettus Bridge and demanding the right to vote, the vicious dogs and even angrier Selma Police insisting they would not—not over their dead bodies.

"Well, I and other marchers were attacked by Bull Connor's dogs. I tried to run and fight them off, but they just kept coming. They tore into my leg and left this bite mark."

He described the pain of being attacked and the anger he felt that after all he'd done for this country, he was not entirely accepted as an American. At that moment, in that hospital room, it became vivid for me. I owed so much to this man and his people for making it possible for me to hold my head high with dignity as a Black physician in the United States. I owed him my best as an oncologist and as a human being.

At the height of the AIDS epidemic, George Washington University was the primary hospital in DC where White HIV-infected patients received care. The virus was mainly infecting and killing young gay men at an unprecedented rate. They came into the hospital with high rates of a lung infection known as *pneumocystis pneumonia*, brain infections such as toxoplasmosis and progressive multifocal leukoencephalopathy (PML), recurrent tuberculosis, and many other opportunistic infections. As a young oncologist in training, I was often consulted because of another consequence of AIDS—Kaposi's sarcoma, which was rare prior to the AIDS epidemic, and non-Hodgkin lymphoma.

But the AIDS crisis was not just impacting White gay men. It was rampant in the Black community as well. Gay men and those who'd become infected due to intravenous drug use and women who'd been sexually infected by the men they loved were also part of this crisis. I'll discuss more about my experience and medical challenges in caring for these men and a few women later.

That's when advancing oncology care through clinical research became a driving passion for me. Through our cancer center, I applied for grants at the intramural, pharmaceutical, and national levels. I collaborated with my PhD colleagues in bench research. I was one of the physicians who investigated through patient chart review whether estrogen replacement in post-menopausal women increased the risk of breast cancer.

During my tenure at Howard, I became interested in cancer risk reduction. Most of my patient care was focused on treating cancer, often advanced stage four disease. But what could be done to reduce the risk of cancer in the first place? We knew there was a cause-and-effect relationship between smoking and lung cancer, among other types of cancer. But what about other cancers like colorectal cancer and breast cancer? Were there also direct causes for these?

> That's when advancing oncology care through clinical research became a driving passion for me.

I was not unique in my questioning. This area was also of great interest to the National Cancer Institute (NCI) and other prominent cancer research organizations. If, through research, we could reduce the risk and increase the lives saved, the cost of care and the emotional trauma it causes could be substantially reduced. In that regard, the NCI sponsored a clinical trial to investigate if tamoxifen, an anti-cancer drug used to treat certain types of breast cancer, could also be used to reduce the *risk* of breast cancer in the first place. The national goal was to recruit more than 11,000 women to the study. Enrollment went well, but the number of African American participants was small.

Howard University Medical Center was approached to help in the effort. The team developed a recruiting strategy that took us into multiple neighborhoods in the DC area; we had discussions with community leaders, visited churches, and had many one-on-one discussions with individuals and families. When the study was completed, the results showed that, indeed, this drug, tamoxifen, did reduce the risk of breast cancer in women who were already at high risk—by almost 50 percent compared to a placebo. Given the challenges of recruiting in this population of predominantly Black women, our efforts were successful. We enrolled the highest number of Black women in the study. Subsequent studies to further understand and improve on these results confirmed that breast cancer risk reduction was indeed possible. The power of clinical research was again evident.

While at Howard, I participated as the co-investigator in the multicenter hemochromatosis and iron overload screening study, or HEIRS for short. This was a multimillion-dollar, National Institute of Health (NIH) funded iron-overload screening study. Complications of iron overload include diabetes mellitus, liver cirrhosis, cardiac diseases, and chronic neurologic disorders. The study investigated the prevalence, genetics, ethnicity, and personal and societal impact of iron overload in the United States and Canada. Mutations in C282Y and H63D genes had been well characterized as the principal genetic defects leading to primary iron overload in people of northern European heritage. However, the prevalence, characterization, and impact on many other ethnic groups was not as well established.

> Subsequent studies to further understand and improve on these results confirmed that breast cancer risk reduction was indeed possible. The power of clinical research was again evident.

The study was of great interest to us because it appeared that, based on some work by Victor Gordeuk at Howard University, iron overload was purported to be caused by a different genetic mutation. But there was no conclusive evidence to support that hypothesis. We also wanted to determine if there was a link between the high prevalence of diabetes in African Americans and iron overload. If the prevalence of iron overload was substantial in African Americans and a clear cause and effect was established, it would be a game changer. Phlebotomy, the standard of care for primary iron overload, could address at least two major health issues and reduce the need for insulin. At least, that was the thinking at the time.

Each research center was charged with recruiting and screening at least two ethnic groups for a total of 20,000 persons per center. Together, the HEIRS goal was ambitious—to screen 100,000 multiethnic persons across the United States. Our center was responsible for enrolling African Americans and Hispanics. Given the historic resistance among African Americans with respect to clinical research, there was great skepticism regarding our ability to enroll 20,000 African Americans and people of Hispanic origins. But under the able leadership of my mentor and friend Dr. Victor Gordeuk, along with a dedicated and focused team that was almost 100 percent Black, we met and exceeded our target ahead of schedule.

Through the power of research, we helped answer several fundamental questions. The most important for our institution was that C282Y and H63D genetic mutations were not a significant issue in African Americans and Hispanics. Therefore, they weren't a major contributor to iron overload and the high rate of diabetes observed in both communities. The HEIRS investigation was conclusive on that question. Thanks to the commitment of Black Americans who worked to recruit Black patients from Black institutions and private offices, we showed that with the correct approach and attitude, research within our community is possible. The leading scientific findings were published in the prestigious *New England Journal of Medicine*.

Some years after my promotion to associate professor, I was asked to head the division of hematology and oncology within the department of medicine. I accepted the new role as interim chief. My responsibility was expanded to include clinical research, patient care, teaching, and, with the appointment, administration. My first response was an emphatic no. The administrative role did not play to my strengths. But I relented and absorbed the added responsibility. There was even more demand on my time during the years that I had a young family to raise.

After fourteen years of serving at the institution—an institution that allowed me to begin to pay a debt of gratitude to a country that has given so much—it was time to go. I left behind colleagues I respected for their clinical acumen, their surgical skills, and their commitment to a venerable institution and all the patients who walked through the door. Freedman's Hospital, which would later become Howard University Hospital, had a legacy of pride and excellence that stretched back to the Civil War. It was an institution that tried mightily to advance a clinical research program, but one in which I had limited success.

I left for reasons so many of my generation of academic clinician-scientists did also: the dwindling grant support for research, increased demand for patient care, less protected time to pursue research, and increased administrative challenges. I left for family and other personal reasons. But in my mind, I was clear about two things: Clinical research in its various forms would be a central part of my career, and I would forever be an advocate for more clinical trials in minority communities. African Americans need to be a part of providing solutions to their health issues, and clinical trials are an essential tool.

I was saddened by the fact that there was such resistance to clinical trials among the Black patients I treated. I understood that the resistance was deeply rooted in the past and the legacy of distrust that still hinders progress today. Tuskegee was still a significant wound in the African American psyche, just like the wound suffered by my patient savaged by Bull Conor's dogs. The wound from Tuskegee and other atrocities committed against Blacks in the name of science and clinical research seemed to be permanent. The gashes and vicious dog bites are still deeply felt in African American communities. It seems that every time the question of a clinical trial is raised, Tuskegee rolls off the tongue.

I want to help change that narrative. I want to tell the story of how, through many Acts of Congress, the efforts of President Bill Clinton, who gave a National Apology for the "sins of Tuskegee," through the actions of international bodies, the clinical trials of the 1930s when the Tuskegee experiment was first started aren't the same now. Clinical trials, in fact, are good medicine.

... the clinical trials of the 1930s when the Tuskegee experiment was first started aren't the same now. Clinical trials, in fact, are good medicine.

Pharmaceuticals

My next stop was the pharmaceutical industry. I stepped into a world to which I previously had only limited exposure. I quickly found out that there was more to this industry than clinical trials. It was an amalgam of science, drug discovery, outsized egos, unmet medical needs, and trial designs. The regulatory demands of the United States Food and Drug Administration (FDA), European Medicines Agency (EMA), and other regulatory bodies were nuanced and demanding.

Having complained bitterly at times about these agencies, I now realized that they were the ultimate gatekeepers. Their standards had to be met and their challenges addressed. For these agencies, safety was the watchword; patient safety now, tomorrow, and always. It was an industry filled with staggering financial risks, as well as the potential for high financial rewards for investors, companies, and individual executives.

From discovery to complete development and approval of one oncology drug, the estimated cost was in the billions of dollars. But on the other hand, if successful, a blockbuster drug could generate more than $2 billion annually. More recent data suggests that in the world of oncology drug development, as little as one in nine drugs receives market approval—that is, approval by a regulatory agency such as the FDA to sell the drug because it has passed regulatory muster.

As I pursued my first job in pharma, a French man and a vice president of a large pharma company in the Philadelphia area casually pointed out that the average cost of a Phase 1 trial at the time would be about $2 million, for which I would be the medical lead. Following that logic with multiple Phase 1, 2, and 3 trials within one company required a magnitude of funding beyond the scope of anything I'd been exposed to before. Two million dollars was small potatoes in the scheme of things. By contrast, if I'd received one-quarter of that amount as an academic, a mere $500,000 to conduct clinical research, I would have been ecstatic.

It's been seventeen years since I left Howard University. Seventeen years since I stepped across a threshold into what some called the dark side of medicine. During these seventeen years, I've had increasing responsibility within the pharmaceutical industry. My time and experience were advantageous at Johnson & Johnson Corporation, first as an associate director of Medical Affairs and then two-plus years later when I transferred to the R&D sector to focus on oncology drug development. Johnson & Johnson was pivotal in helping me understand the multiple roles a physician plays in the industry, but after eight years, it was time to move on.

My next stop was Incyte Corporation in Wilmington, Delaware, where I was hired as the executive director. The first oncology trial I led was a Phase 3 trial in metastatic cancer of the pancreas. It did not go well. After strenuous efforts by myself and the team—including multiple visits to research physicians in Germany, France, Denmark, Sweden, and clinicians in the US—the trial was a failure.

Multiple trials and meetings later, I was asked to lead a Phase 2 trial in patients diagnosed with acute graph versus host disease (AGVD) and a Phase 3 trial in cGVHD. The two diseases are different in many ways but have overlapping symptoms. Both diseases are the result of bone marrow transplants, a treatment given to patients with bone marrow diseases such as leukemia, lymphoma, or multiple myeloma. After multiple chemotherapy treatments have failed to cure these diseases, the doctor may decide that the best hope for the patient is a bone marrow transplant. If the patient agrees, the medical team will preferably find a close family member like a sibling or parent whose blood cells are a match. The relative's bone cells are hopefully genetically close enough to the patient's that it will graph into the host without too many complications. But no matter how closely matched, there are always some complications where the cells from the relative (graph) attack the skin, liver, gut, and bone marrow of the host. The effect amounts to the transplanted cells (the graph) rejecting the host cells. In other words the graph cells now treat the host as the *foreigner* and tries to get rid of it. Something needs to be done for the host to reduce the rate of rejection from the graph.

After enrolling seventy patients, our Phase 2 trial in AGVHD was approved. The first of its kind, Phase 2 enrolled only seventy patients. US FDA wanted to be sure the company didn't just get lucky with such a small number of patients. So, the confirmatory Phase 3 trial in AGVHD took a longer time and required more patients. The US FDA also approved it, but that was after I left the company. The results of the Phase 3 confirmed the success we saw in the Phase 2.

Perhaps one of my proudest moments was leading a Phase 1 trial for sickle cell disease, one that I campaigned for and received. Unfortunately, the drug was found to be too toxic, and the study was stopped. No one died as a result.

The one constant has always been the patient and their safety. Ensuring that they met the criterion as outlined in the protocol, ensuring that the informed consent form (ICF) provided the necessary information with sufficient clarity, so the patients could truly make an *informed* decision. The signed-by-the-patient form serves to protect the rights, dignity, and autonomy of the patient from being violated, rights that were totally discarded during the syphilis experiments at Tuskegee. Nobody who agrees to participate in a clinical trial should be uninformed about the risks and potential benefits—or the potential that they may not benefit. Clinical trials are entirely voluntary, and they sometimes save the patient's life.

> Perhaps one of my proudest moments was leading a Phase 1 trial for sickle cell disease . . .

What troubles me was how difficult it was to enroll Black patients in any clinical trial that I led. Of course, since I no longer had direct responsibility for patients, participation was left to the patient's treating physicians and team. However, over time, I noted a gradual shift in the attitude that some pharmaceutical and biotech companies' leadership had toward sensitivities around this issue. For some there was more in the research budget and more resources dedicated to recruiting and retaining a more diverse population to clinical trials. There was an increased demand from the US FDA, multiple national medical institutions, Black church ministers, and others that trials needed to be more inclusive. The current health disparity is a national blight and a widening chasm. Clinical trials that end on a positive note can narrow that gap.

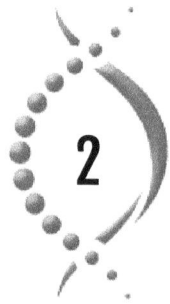

NEVER FORGET: TUSKEGEE AND HENRIETTA LACKS

"Unbeknownst to her, the doctor had already lost our trust. She hadn't explained my mother's diagnosis or prognosis as she had promised. . . Instead, she asked my mother to donate her time and possibly risk her health and life for science. Nothing had been done to address my mother's fears about her disease, its treatment, or her own mortality."

—*New England Journal of Medicine, August 29, 2019*

D epression-era 1930s United States, WW I, or the Great War as it was known then, had already concluded by 1918; the Spanish flu pandemic had dissipated, the Roaring Twenties came to a screeching halt, and now it was time to pay the piper. The Depression brought misery and mass internal migration. Wall Street crashed and with it dragged many to death by suicide, long food lines, and tent cities. Thus was the impact on the majority of White Americans. Most Black Americans fared far worse.

In Tuskegee, a small rural town nestled in Alabama, the plight of poor Black people, many of whom were sharecroppers and most of them illiterate, was dismal. If many of their White neighbors couldn't feed and clothe their own, how would they? Cotton was a major commodity and a staple crop for sharecroppers. In 1929, it sold for thirty-five cents per pound. Due to a variety of factors, the price fell even further to five cents per pound by 1935.

Some left farming to pursue industrial jobs. But the night of the Great Depression overshadowed them there, too. Many lost their jobs. Consequently, many had little to eat, and for some, milk powder was their only daily meal. A perfect storm was brewing.

Amid this ongoing economic meltdown, *opportunity* knocked for six hundred Black men. The federal government made an offer to four hundred men diagnosed with "bad blood" and two hundred without. Based on the CDC's account, in exchange for their participation in the United States Public Health Service Syphilis Study at Tuskegee (the Tuskegee experiment), the men would receive free medical examinations, free meals, and burial insurance—a chance to have some dignity in death. Federal government-sponsored researchers collaborated with White physicians in Alabama to conduct the study. Of course, they could be trusted to do the right thing, or so the victims thought. Evil often lurks where there is ignorance, disinformation, and unwillingness to ask the right questions or know what the right questions are.

The lie had been cast. The men were told their bad blood, which included anemia, syphilis, and fatigue, would be treated if they agreed to participate in the study. Even more galling and to further sell the lie, the experiment was conducted at the venerable Tuskegee Institute founded by the august Black scholar Booker T. Washington, a cynical method that gave the study a further air of credibility. In Depression-era Black Alabama, accessing food was a high priority. Medicine, if you could afford it, was a luxury. Six hundred men agreed to participate. The benefits seemed to be a no-brainer.

At best, according to some reports, bad blood was treated only with painkillers such as aspirin. The primary focus of the researchers, and by extension the federal government because they were the sponsors/funders of the study, was to conduct an observation study to document the natural history of syphilis compared to uninfected men, but with no intervention, without treatment. No informed consent was requested, and thus, no informed consent form (ICF) was signed by participants. The signed informed consent form is a required legal document today that recognizes the rights of the patient or participant in any human research and spells out its purpose, procedures, duration, potential risks, and definitive statements that a positive outcome can't be guaranteed. No such document existed at the time.

The men were told several lies:

Lie #1: No treatment was intended.

Lie #2: In 1932, there was no known effective treatment for syphilis.

Lie #3: If treatment was available, it was not intended for this group of men.

Lie #4: The true purpose of the experiment was not stated—at least not to the participants.

There is a long and painful history of medical experimentation conducted in the name of science in the US and other countries. There are abundant cases of grave robbing where corpses were dug up and peddled as cadavers used to teach medical students gross anatomy. Army psychedelic drug experiments were conducted on unsuspecting soldiers in the US Army, to name a few. The Tuskegee experiment was another in the string of such abuses and everyday atrocities in the name of medical science and national interests. This was the medical power dynamic on full display; it was an acceptable behavior

There is a long and painful history of medical experimentation conducted in the name of science in the US and other countries.

at the time that few challenged. This was an abuse of patient rights.

But there were a few brave people who questioned the merits and the science of this experiment. As early as the 1960s, Public Health employees such as Peter Buxtun and others began to question the study design and ethics of the experiment. As reported, he filed an official protest with his employer, the United States Public Health Services, in 1966, thirty-two years after the start of the experiment. But his concerns fell on deaf ears. He persisted, and in 1968, he filed another protest with the same results. No one listened. As he saw it, the longstanding experiment was unethical, and participation lacked transparency regarding what the experiment entailed. Therefore, the men were being "duped" for more than thirty years in a poorly designed study that lacked scientific merit. But medical science had to be served; there were scientific papers to be written and careers to be advanced.

Finally, an Associated Press reporter broke the story in 1972, some forty years later. What followed were the expected recriminations and finger-pointing. But the damage had been done. And because untreated syphilis progresses, the damage to these men's health continued. Many men died. By 1972, only seventy-four men were alive. On May 16, 1997, two-and-one-half decades from termination and more than half a century from the beginning of the experiment, President Bill Clinton issued a National Apology. In the East Room of the

White House with surviving relatives in attendance, he said in part:

> The White House is the people's house . . . The eight men who are survivors of the syphilis study at Tuskegee are a living link to a time not so very long ago that many Americans would prefer not to remember, but we dare not forget. It was a time when our nation failed to live up to its ideals, when our nation broke the trust with our people that is the very foundation of our democracy. It isn't only in remembering that shameful past that we can make amends and repair our nation, but it is in remembering that past that we can build a better present and a better future. And without remembering it, we cannot make amends, and we cannot go forward.
>
> So today, America does remember the hundreds of men used in research without their knowledge and consent. We remember them and their family members. Men who were poor and African American, without resources and with few alternatives, they believed they had found hope when they were offered free medical care by the United States Public Health Service. They were betrayed. Medical people are supposed to help when we need care, but even once a cure was discovered, they were denied help, and they were lied to by their government. Our government is supposed to protect the rights of its citizens; their rights were trampled upon. Forty years, hundreds of men betrayed, along with their wives and children, along with the community in Macon County, Alabama, the City of Tuskegee, the fine university there, and the larger African American community.
>
> The United States government did something that was wrong—deeply, profoundly, morally wrong. It was an outrage to our commitment to integrity and equality for all our citizens.

To the survivors, to the wives and family members, the children, and the grandchildren, I say what you know: No power on Earth can give you back the lives lost, the pain suffered, the years of internal torment and anguish. What was done cannot be undone. But we can end the silence. We can stop turning our heads away. We can look at you in the eye and finally say on behalf of the American people, what the United States government did was shameful, and I'm sorry.

The American people are sorry—for the loss, for the years of hurt. You did nothing wrong, but you were grievously wronged. I apologize, and I'm sorry that this apology has been so long in coming.

Patients' Rights

One of the many changes that came of Tuskegee is patients' rights and the high ethical standard required of any organization, university, or pharmaceutical company that conducts clinical trials. Through an Act of Congress, The US government authorized the National Commission for the Protection of Human Subjects of Biomedical and Behavioral Research, which was created to investigate and then recommend necessary changes and improvements to human research in the United States. After four years of meetings, the Belmont Report, a watershed in human subjects' research, was issued in 1976. It issued three basic principles:

1. Respect for the rights of each person: This principle points out the rights of *the person* first and not just the rights of *a patient.*
2. Beneficence: The welfare of the person should be the optimal goal of any human subject research. That should be the first consideration while reducing the risk of harm to each participant. This is closely aligned

with the Latin medical dictum *primum non nochere,* or *above all, do no harm.*

3. Justice: Decisions made to include or exclude a person for clinical studies should be made fairly and without personal or scientific bias.

One of the practical applications of the Belmont Report was the requirement of a signed informed consent form (ICF). ICFs vary by study and each study's complexity, the institution where the trial is conducted, the length of the study, and the disease to be studied. The FDA requires eight critical elements for an acceptable ICF:

1. Description of the clinical investigation
2. Risks and discomforts
3. Benefits
4. Alternative procedures or treatment
5. Confidentiality
6. Compensation and medical treatment in the event of injury
7. Contacts
8. Voluntary participation

Another primary recommendation of the Belmont Report requires all study protocols to be critiqued by an institutional review board (or IRB), also known as the Ethics Committee in the European Union and the United Kingdom. According to the FDA, the primary goal and purpose of an IRB is to "approve, require modifications in (to secure approval), or disapprove research. This group review serves an important role in the protection of the rights and welfare of human research subjects."

There are additional protections in place that focus on patients' rights and protection. The US FDA encourages all sponsors of clinical trials to begin a dialogue with patients, starting with the proposed drug and what is known about its safety in animals, the proposed design of the study, the population to be studied, and what safety measures will be in place to protect the rights of the patient. The dialogue is encouraged at every step, from Phase 1 up until Phase 3 is completed and the sponsor believes the drug is ready for approval.

Another critical requirement is that all studies conducted in the US or any sponsor outside the US who hopes to get approval must register their study on the government website ClinicalTrials.gov. Patients and their families or any other interested party have free access to this information. Some patients have moved across state lines or traveled internationally to access some of these trials. World-renowned medical centers, such as MD Anderson Cancer Center in Houston, Texas, and the Mayo Clinic in Rochester, Minnesota, draw patients from all over the world—the Middle East, Africa, Asia, and Europe. Clinical trials provide excellent medical care. Some have said they received better care, have a greater understanding of their disease, received treatment when nothing else was available, and they often believe they are paying it forward.

AND THEN THERE'S MRS. HENRIETTA LACKS, whose experience at the hands of a world-renowned academic center is a different version of what happened at Tuskegee. Rebecca Skloot, an award-winning science reporter for the *New York Times*, tells Mrs. Lacks's story, which took place more than fifty years ago, in her book *The Immortal Life of Henrietta Lacks*. It's the story of a poor and disrespected Black woman. This story has garnered national and international attention and has been retold through interviews, talk shows, and an HBO documentary produced by Oprah Winfrey and Alan Ball.

The story begins in the 1950s when Mrs. Lacks was in her thirties—a full twenty years after the start of the Tuskegee experiment. At the heart of this painful history is the disrespect shown for the rights, opinions, and wishes of Mrs. Lacks and her family. This was about control of one's body, and who makes or is authorized to make decisions for that body and what happens to it. Ignoring her rights and experimenting on her cervical cancer tissue against her wishes, however noble, was essentially saying, "Your rights and freedoms do not matter. Medical science can do what it wishes, and there's nothing you can do about it." We know that during this era, many unethical human studies were being conducted at some of the most prestigious institutions throughout the country. First, the surgeon at Johns Hopkins Hospital informed her and her husband that they wanted to use her cells for future research. Skloot reports that although her husband was informed, he made it clear to the doctor that he did not consent to having his wife's cancer cells used in experiments. By ethical standards, nothing more should have come of it.

Despite the family's refusal, the surgeon collected cells for experimentation anyway. The cells were then replicated and commercialized to the tune of millions of dollars. The family was the last to know. Johns Hopkins Hospital in Baltimore, Maryland, disputes the details of Mrs. Lacks's story. But her story overlaps with what happened at Tuskegee, which was a very permissive time in human clinical experimentation. It was fertile ground for this level of abuse and disrespect.

Had Mrs. Lacks lived, she would be more than 100 years old. Advanced-stage cervical cancer was incurable in the mid-1950s. Her immortalized cells live on and have become a building block that advanced the clinical science of cancer, the polio vaccine, and genome mapping, to name a few. In a recognition of Mrs. Lacks and the HeLa cells' contribution to science, the Johns Hopkins University wrote:

Among the important scientific discoveries of the last century was the first immortal human cell line known as "HeLa"—a remarkably durable and prolific line of cells obtained during the treatment of Henrietta's cancer by Johns Hopkins researcher Dr. George Gey in 1951.

Although these were the first cells that could be easily shared and multiplied in a lab setting, Johns Hopkins has never sold or profited from the discovery or distribution of HeLa cells and does not own the rights to the HeLa cell line. Rather, Johns Hopkins offered HeLa cells freely and widely for scientific research.

Over the past several decades, this cell line has contributed to many medical breakthroughs, from research on the effects of zero gravity in outer space and the development of polio and COVID-19 vaccines, to the study of leukemia, the AIDS virus, and cancer worldwide.

Although many other cell lines are in use today, HeLa cells have supported advances in most fields of medical research in the years since HeLa cells were isolated. On the face of it, having access to these cells and the outstanding research and the benefit to humanity that resulted, is a tribute to these scientists. Unfortunate as the sequence of events was, the positive impact on society is incalculable. And for that, we owe Mrs. Lacks a debt of gratitude.

But things have changed since that time. In my experience, the most significant emphasis has been and always will be to outline the medical risks and prioritize patient safety above all else. As an executive in the drug development industry, I have seen and attended countless internal meetings and meetings with regulatory authorities, been in protracted discussions with laboratory scientists to further enhance patients' safety, building on what we know about animal experiments, and have attended meetings with external scientific and medical experts before, during, and after a clinical trial is conducted. We do it all in the name of safety, robust informed consent, and the quality of the science. The report also requires that the population of patients selected for study is based on fairness, and they must be protected against discrimination or selection bias based on things like race, gender, zip code, or ethnicity, among other things.

The Belmont Report was pivotal in establishing an enhanced, nationwide bioethical standard of human research. It was a watershed moment in the interest of patient rights, safety, and protection. In its own words, the US Health and Human Services, Office of Human Protection, the Belmont Report was:

> . . . written by the National Commission for the Protection of Human Subjects of Biomedical and Behavioral Research. The Commission, created as a result of the National Research Act of 1974, was charged with identifying the basic ethical principles that should underlie the conduct of biomedical and behavioral research involving human subjects and developing guidelines to assure that such research is conducted in accordance with those principles . . . the Commission published the Belmont Report, which identifies basic ethical principles and guidelines that address ethical issues arising from the conduct of research with human subjects.

Since then, there have been specific reports related to research on fetuses and research involving prisoners, children, and others.

A few years ago, one of the companies I worked for conducted a clinical trial related to a hematologic disease. We had difficulty enrolling patients, so I visited a site in my capacity as the lead study physician where all indications were that the university that agreed to participate should be able to enroll at a better rate. The study investigator at the university and I met to discuss how we could help move things forward.

She acknowledged that, indeed, there was a high volume of patients they cared for at her site. But she said that perhaps 50 percent of these potential study patients came from the nearby long-term penitentiary. The university was the sole provider of care for prisoners diagnosed with cancer who could potentially benefit from a bone marrow transplant and the management of its complications. Based on the vigilance of the physician-scientist, it became clear to me that enrolling prisoners, no matter how much they could advance our study, was off-limits. I knew this from my prior experiences, but at that moment, in a dramatic way, it was evident that the Belmont Report had taken hold in that academic center.

One of the striking ironies of the Belmont Report is that the very guardrails put in place, triggered in no small part by Tuskegee to ensure the human rights of African Americans, have led to the unintended consequence of further distrust of clinical trials, not less. So many remain gun-shy of "the system." On the other hand, others have armed themselves with the right to participate, ask questions, inform themselves, and seek redress if their rights are violated. If there is abuse and violation of rights, there is also redress through legal means.

> . . . President Clinton's apology on behalf of the nation was a good and sincere start.

Yes, President Clinton's apology on behalf of the nation was a good and sincere start. Pharmaceutical companies are now coming forward and acknowledging that there were abuses, expressing an appreciation that African Americans have unique challenges participating in trials, and are taking multiple steps to make amends.

The advances in cancer research and the benefits to the American public over the last fifty years have been breathtaking! Many of the advances have come because of the federal government funding through the NCI and to the NIH in general. Funding has come through taxpayer dollars. Life expectancy after a cancer diagnosis has increased, and the cancer incidence has decreased.

In my opinion, it would be a shame if African Americans, who are equal shareholders in government spending, do not take full advantage. We know that biotech companies and the pharmaceutical industry have taken basic research and early clinical trials and turbocharged them into medicines that are good for the public. However, African Americans lag in almost every cancer statistic: cancer prevalence, cancer survival rates, and treatment outcomes, among others. To be sure, the determinants of health and cancer health outcomes aren't driven by clinical trials alone. Much more has been done to reduce the incidence of cancer through cancer screening and educating the public regarding smoking, for example.

The naysayers who criticize the War on Cancer strategy that began in 1971 are correct. Even more needs to be done to reduce the incidence of cancer. Unfortunately, cancer will occur in some, even with the best cancer reduction strategies. However, clinical trials can play a significant role in prolonging survival. Many of the advances in clinical medicine are the result of the brave patients who volunteer, brilliant scientists, and compassionate clinical investigators who are committed in their unique way to uplifting patients and our society.

Despite the justified anger and the pain we still feel from the past, we can move forward as a people in a system that seems to lock us out. But for our sake and that of our children, we should not keep ourselves locked in by our fears and misgivings. Armed with knowledge, bioethical guidelines, and the knowledge that there are advocates within and outside the medical system, African Americans have and must continue to demand more participation in clinical research focused on their medical needs and interests.

We know the past can't be rewritten; many have tried and failed. But they can pay it forward. Advocating for better trial designs, participating in available clinical trials, and

> Despite the justified anger and the pain we still feel from the past, we can move forward as a people in a system that seems to lock us out.

supporting STEM education for our children is a start. Our children will become biomedical scientists, epidemiologists, physicians, and industry leaders who not only have a seat at the table but also sit at the head of the table.

Yes, there has been abuse. Yes, there is justifiable anger. But unless we move beyond these many pain points, African Americans will be looking back in anger in another fifty years, wondering why more wasn't done to advance their health. We must train the next generation of clinical trialists who look like the people they serve and hope to attract to clinical trials. The data is clear that there is a greater level of trust when that is done.

3

WHAT IS A CLINICAL TRIAL?

*"Change won't come if we wait for some other person or some
other time. We are the ones we've been waiting for.
We are the change that we seek."*

—President Barak Obama

He walked into the office. I took one look at him, and I could tell, as an oncologist, that his cancer was advanced. He was jaundiced, his clothes hung on him like a skeleton, and he had a massive belly.

"Mr. MP, I want to talk to you about your diagnosis," I said. He was a Black man of average height, soft-spoken, and he'd worked hard all his life to support his wife and children. Now he was in trouble. He had an aggressive cancer that threatened to destroy the very life he'd worked so hard to build.

He was referred by the hospital's surgical team with an established diagnosis of metastatic pancreas cancer. They correctly concluded that he was inoperable. Since surgery was not an option, a chemotherapy regimen was the next best option for him at the time. However, even the best available chemotherapy regimen was not a promising approach because treatment often fails for a patient with metastatic-stage 4 disease.

"I want to discuss cancer treatment options with you," I continued, "but the best available and approved treatment isn't very effective for people with cancer of the pancreas. Only a few respond to chemotherapy, and if they do, it's only for a short while. The prognosis isn't very good, so I want to suggest the possibility of a clinical trial," I explained. "There's no guarantee, but I think it may give you a better shot."

The US FDA had just approved gemcitabine as a treatment for cancer of the pancreas. Still, the data supporting the approval was met with skepticism by some in the medical oncology community. The initial approval was not because of an improvement in survival. It was based on the evidence that quality of life was improved with this regimen. Follow-up studies with gemcitabine for advanced cancer of the pancreas did lead to improved survival.

These were desperate times for patients with this aggressive disease. It's a cancer that seems to gobble up and destroy one organ after the other in rapid succession. Despite the best medical and scientific minds, millions of dollars of research, and keen public advocacy, there had been no significant improvements until some years after I last took care of Mr. MP. It was one of the most disheartening cancers to manage as an oncologist. I, like some other oncologists, often felt like a failure because the treatment options were so ineffective. This sometimes overwhelming sense of failure and the lack of rapid advances in cancer management inspired us to seek answers, to work harder, and to leave behind a legacy of success.

Mr. MP respectfully heard me out, as so many patients do when meeting with the doctor. He nodded to indicate that he understood as I outlined the reasons and the potential benefits of a clinical trial. He also understood that the final decision was his.

His final comment was summed up in one phrase: "Well, doc, I don't want to be a guinea pig. If the regular treatment doesn't work for anyone else, it will work for me."

That phrase, "guinea pig," captured what I'd heard so many times and in other ways from so many of my patients as it related to clinical trials. I thought it was a fear of the unknown. Clinical trials, after all, are experiments designed to find a better way to treat patients. Or was he expressing his distrust of the medical system, questions about my true motive for offering a trial (*Is the doctor making money off me if I participate?*), or most importantly, was it that he didn't understand what takes place during a clinical trial? I also thought he could mean, "I remember Tuskegee, and I know what happened there."

Defining and educating cancer patients about clinical trials—the benefits, the risks, and the guardrails that are now in place—is critical if we are to lower the walls of distrust, fear, and hostility. It will take time, but we must work at warp speed.

Physicians themselves are vital to the recruiting process because in order to participate in the trial, they must first gain the patient's trust. Some studies have confirmed that patients are more likely to participate in a trial if one is being conducted in their physician's office. On the other hand, the same patient will think twice if they have to go to another doctor for the same trial. Patients are also more open to a trial if someone of the same race or ethnicity and background conducts it.

Patient-by-patient, one clinical trial at a time, investigators must demonstrate basic competence with respect to Black patients' historical health context. They must be sensitive about why there's been historically low enrollment among African Americans. The good news is that medical centers, government agencies, and the pharmaceutical industry are more aware of this and are beginning to turn the ship. But it's like turning an aircraft carrier in the ocean. It's a massive effort and takes time, but it can be steered in the right direction.

The "guinea pig syndrome" is a real thing among Black *and* White patients. A few years ago, Gwendolyn P. Quinn and colleagues explored this phenomenon based on a survey, and they published their findings in "The Guinea Pig Syndrome: Improving Clinical Trial Participation Among Thoracic Patients" in the *Journal of Thoracic Oncology*. She and her colleagues examined "lung cancer patients' knowledge, attitudes, and behavior regarding clinical trials and to develop an effective intervention for increasing patient knowledge and awareness of clinical trials for lung cancer patients."

The NCI keeps a database that tracks and documents cancer statistics reports showing that despite declining cancer rates, Black men and women together have the highest rate of lung cancer than any other racial group and the highest lung-cancer-specific mortality. This is true even though we know that on a population basis, there are more White smokers than Blacks.

I gave a lung cancer presentation to a nurse's group some time ago. In my preparation, I found some disturbing data that may help explain these high rates among African Americans. It appears that the carcinogens inhaled with smoking are cleared at a slower rate, and they linger in the body for a longer time among African

> ... Black men and women together have the highest rate of lung cancer than any other racial group and the highest lung-cancer-specific mortality.

American participants. Prolonged exposure increases the potential carcinogenic effects on lung tissue, as well as other smoking-related tissue, such as the bladder. So, even when the individual may smoke fewer cigarettes per day, there isn't a proportionately lower concentration of carcinogens.

Part of my presentation included a slide of a Kool cigarette advertisement on the back of a trendy magazine whose readership was mainly Black. It was a scene of young, handsome, energetic, carefree, and upwardly mobile African Americans on a beach somewhere in the Caribbean. Professor Keith Wailoo, of Princeton University recently published an inciteful book, *Pushing Cool: Big Tobacco, Racial Marketing, and the Untold Story of Menthol Cigarette.* In it, he says, "A lot of Black periodicals, like Ebony, became so dependent on tobacco advertising that they were silent of the devastating impact of smoking in the Black community." Wailoo's research documents a toxic brew of tobacco marketing skills, bolstered with the help of social scientists and psychologists—and aided by Black civic organizations and politicians. This led to high profit margins for the companies but reaped a grim harvest of lung and other tobacco-related cancers in Black communities.

In Gwendolyn Quinn's survey, only 10 percent of a total of forty-three participants were Black; the rest were White. We can only speculate why the percentage of participating Blacks was so low. Some of the responses showed that patients feared being guinea pigs and had a belief that if a trial was offered, it was the last ditch, and all hope was gone. Quinn said that misunderstanding the purpose of a clinical trial was very high among both new and existing patients.

On the other hand, patients who had previously participated in a trial had very different attitudes. Their position was primarily positive and more trusting. They'd already leaped and had realized the potential benefits of a clinical trial: clinical trials "equate with good medicine." Thankfully, some Blacks participated, but the percentage was too low to derive meaningful conclusions about their attitudes toward clinical trials.

Misunderstanding of clinical trials is high across the US population and may explain the low overall participation when compared to patients in the European Union and the United

Kingdom. These concerns are exceptionally high in the Black community. But it's even further heightened because of what happened at Tuskegee and other blatant acts of racism under the guise of human research.

Kiameesha R. Evans and colleagues captured this very well in "The Role of Health Literacy on African American and Hispanic/Latino Perspectives on Cancer Clinical Trials," published in the *Journal of Cancer Education* in 2012. Focus groups were formed, and a series of questions were posed. Here are some of the questions:

- What do you think the benefits of cancer clinical trials are?
- Do you think that something like Tuskegee could still happen today?
- This may be difficult to imagine, but if you had cancer, do you think you would participate in a treatment trial?
- What would it depend on?
- Some African Americans/Hispanics say they might participate in a clinical cancer study if the researcher or the people who recruited them were African American/ Hispanic; would that be true in your case?

These questions get to the heart of the fear of clinical trials among many Black patients. Here's a telling response to the question of the ethnicity of the treating physician in Evans's paper: "I don't think that it should make a difference what color a person . . . is, but realistically, most people are comfortable dealing with their own ethnic group." Those in the scientific and clinical research community have heard this statement in more ways than one. Patients are more likely to participate in clinical trials based on the trust and confidence they have in the practitioners and the institution where they receive care.

In the hematology and medical oncology community, less than 10 percent are African Americans, and even fewer are trained as clinical trialists. That won't cut it.

Some drug companies and organizations are trying to fix the shortage of minority clinical trialists. Take, for example, the programs kicked off in 2019 by the US FDA known as Project Socrates, which was focused on "building an educational network" that bridges oncology drug development and regulatory sciences. Under the Socrates umbrella are opportunities to expose high school students and recent high school graduates from underrepresented and underserved communities to drug development. This ongoing program has already trained over seventy students, and it will take time to bear fruit. To address the more immediate need, the FDA collaborated with the American Association of Cancer Research (AACR). At the height of the COVID-19 pandemic in 2020, they launched another training program. This time, it was aimed at MDs, MD-PhDs, and DOs to educate them further on what's essential in oncology drug development: the importance and benefit of enrolling diverse patients in clinical trials, data integrity and collection, and the importance of monitoring drug safety. More companies need to follow the US FDA and AACR lead.

They also found that there was limited and incorrect understanding of scientific information and perceptions of clinical trials, as well as trust issues, as exemplified in the statement, "I don't wanna be a guinea pig either. I don't want you to give me something and then say, well, this might, you know, I don't know how it's gonna affect you. This might do this; I can't really say. You know doctors always say that." Taken together, Evans's findings were almost identical to the responses in the Quinn survey, which, again, was comprised of 93 percent White patients. Just as interesting, she also noted there's a strong dependency on home remedies among some participants, which are not effective.

This last point struck a nerve for me. In my practice, I've had long conversations with patients who, in the rejection of the Western approach to practicing medicine, happily extolled the benefits of herbal and "natural" medicines. At the same time, many of these patients are convinced that the modern approach to medical care is driven only by a profit motive. I've had at least one patient frustrated with the side effects of chemotherapy reject further treatment and decide to take Laetrile.

"Laetrile," she said, "is natural. I have done my research, and there is lots of evidence to show that it is very effective against cancer."

I was pretty aware of the Laetrile phenomenon and the heavy marketing campaign by some medical establishments in Mexico that tout the cancer benefits of Laetrile.

"So, what evidence do you have that Laetrile is effective against cancer?" I asked.

"There are lots of testimonials in magazines and online where patients say that they have been helped. I am willing to take my chances," she said.

"How will you pay for the treatment?" I asked. "Is it covered by insurance?" I knew full well that it was not.

She told me that she was willing to do whatever it took to get the treatment.

There was no scientific evidence, no verifiable data, to support Laetrile as an effective cancer treatment. Some have labeled it the equivalent of snake oil or quackery. The Laetrile cancer story has been around for a long time. Laetrile is not approved and is banned for human use by US FDA. Far from being a cure, it has led to cyanide poisoning and other side effects in some patients. Laetrile is just one of many examples of how some alternate cancer treatments can cause harm because time is lost and the cancer progresses, even while ineffective, fake medicine is administered.

Others didn't totally reject the Western approach, but they either secretly or overtly combined the best of the West with remedies based on ancient practices and recommendations from naturalists. The best minds in the medical, psychological, and social sciences will need more potent remedies and better antidotes to overcome these decades-long fears and pain points that have plagued our community. We must give communities of color a reason to believe, lower their guard, and begin to reap the benefits that they so richly deserve, but many deny themselves. It will take time. But a hyperfocus on these persistent issues is as important as the spark that lit the fuse for the War on Cancer some fifty years ago.

The Tuskegee experiment was not a clinical trial. That is not how things are done today. Clinical trials, if successful, bring hope to patients. They lift the human spirit. They offer the possibility of new drugs and new treatments to relieve the physical suffering of humanity, one disease at a time. Success requires the informed, voluntary cooperation of patients to provide answers—answers to often tricky and perplexing medical questions. Transparently, they can provide answers for the living and future generations.

> The Tuskegee experiment was not a clinical trial. That is not how things are done today.

Clinical trials pull patients into new conversations about themselves, their health needs, and their future. Any trial should always be and *is* about patients and *their* needs. Patients seek the help and advice of doctors and expect them to provide objective diagnoses and prescribe the correct therapy where needed. Sometimes, these remedies are not equally effective for all patients with the same disease. Sometimes, medications work on a limited basis. New ones must be prescribed to treat "old mangy dogs." Sometimes, we need new tricks for persistent enemies.

At times, suffering cannot be relieved because new and better treatments are not available. The same cancer treated two years ago may come back with a vengeance. The new or recurring cancer cells now have slightly different biologies or characteristics that make them resistant to prior therapies, hence the phrase "the changing face of cancer." This is very often the case with patients diagnosed with advanced or metastatic cancers. A particular cancer may respond for a while and then develop resistance to the treatment. In some ways, this is no different from a patient with uncontrolled high blood pressure. The first treatment may have started with one effective drug, but over time, the blood pressure may become worse, and the doctor has to either change to a new drug or add to the existing one to achieve better control. If no new drug is available, a patient will most likely continue to deteriorate from ravaging and progressive cancer. *Progressive* is an unfortunate term because it means the cancer is worse, not better. When these changes occur (and they sometimes do), it's an opportunity for patients, doctors, and the industry to form partnerships against the specific cancer to find new treatments.

We know significant advances are happening, which is one reason for the improvement in cancer survival for Americans. New drugs are developed every day, and the public, perhaps through public campaigns, needs to know how hard their tax dollars result in dividends for them. Some think that as industry and government agencies share more with the public, the barriers that lead to mistrust will decrease. In other words, openness builds trust.

Patient education is vital if more patients are to move away from guinea pig syndrome and on to full participation. Clinical research and clinical trials are for the benefit of human beings and a better society.

Before *clinical* comes *pre-clinical,* which utilizes various methods to characterize and better understand new molecules that could become anticancer agents or assess existing drugs that are redirected to manage an old cancer problem. This is the actual guinea pig stage, where scientists test the effects of drugs on animals: mice, monkeys, and, yes, guinea pigs, and even a species of miniature pigs known as mini-pigs. Every effort is made to understand as much as possible regarding the effects of a new drug and how it may impact human lives, such as its side effects and the effects it has on the organs such as the liver, kidney, heart, and lungs. Furthermore, does the drug shrink tumors in animals? There are even computer models used to evaluate the potential drug effects.

> Clinical research and clinical trials are for the benefit of human beings and a better society.

The effects on animals that were produced under scientific conditions are then shared and discussed with a medical team. If the results are encouraging, the medical team will begin a rigorous process of testing the drug in human beings, starting with a Phase 1 study. It is never that straightforward, but the focus is on how to make the drug as safe as possible for the next step.

Drug studies done first in animals are good but not sufficient to be administered to large groups of patients. There is a step-by-step process whereby clinical researchers take the next step to move from animal testing to testing on human beings. We go through a series of steps starting with Phase 1, or first-in-human trial, where the first consideration is the safety of patients, how the body breaks down the molecule, how the molecule is removed from the body, and what may be a safe dose to be administered to a larger group of patients. With a good understanding of what a safe dose may be, we then move to Phase 2, where safety again remains the number one concern, but now we are testing to see if the drug is both safe *and* shows signs of being effective. Phase 3 requires more patients than Phase 1 and Phase 2. Depending on the disease being studied and guidance from regulatory bodies such as the US FDA, it may range from a few hundred to thousands of patients. We can transition to Phase 3, the so-called randomized control trial design, because there's strong proof of safety and some proof that the drug will work for the unmet medical need being studied. Yes, it is medical science. We are trying to answer clinical questions through scientific methods. In Phase 3, studies are randomized, meaning that the new molecules we will call Drug A after testing in Phase 1 and Phase 2 are now randomly compared to Drug B. Some patients will receive Drug A and others Drug B. What we want to know with this randomization is if Drug A will be better than Drug B to either cure this cancer or make the patient live longer or better with treatment.

Even after Phase 1 and Phase 2 trials, there's no guarantee that Drug A will be more effective than Drug B. There are still uncertainties. There are still risks. So even if a patient gets Drug A, there's no guarantee of a positive outcome.

Clinical trials drive drug development and, ultimately, better clinical outcomes through new medications. Many patients find them complex and confusing. Sometimes, the goals for Phase 1 trials aren't clear to patients. If they agree to go forward as participants, doctors need to make it clear that the first goal is to understand how the drug works in human beings, to understand how toxic it is, and to find a safe dose that can be carried forward into Phase 2. Patients also need to know that they may not personally get any benefit from the drug. In other words, doctors should not offer patients unrealistic expectations for the drug.

That said, Dr. Takebe of the NCI said in a 2022 interview that in the past, only about 4 to 5 percent of Phase 1 participants received some clinical benefit. "But we and others have now shown that things have changed. Participating in Phase 1 trials has more potential for clinical benefit than is commonly believed, largely due to the development of modern cancer drugs, like targeted therapies, immunotherapies, and new combination therapies," she says. On the other hand, some patients think it's better to avoid clinical studies altogether and let someone else do the heavy lifting.

> Clinical trials drive drug development and, ultimately, better clinical outcomes through new medications.

But in a recent survey published in the *Clinical Journal of Oncology Nursing*, a more realistic picture emerges. The article points out that most patients participated because they were encouraged by their physician, were altruistic, and expected to achieve a more stable disease and better quality of life. They concluded that "patients participating in Phase 1 trials remain optimistic about treatment options while aware of their mortality."

A Phase 1 trial is clinical science's method of answering some basic questions about a new drug or one that is being clinically repurposed. The drug has already been extensively tested in animals, so the Phase 1 clinical trialist asks:

- What is the correct starting dose in humans?
- How safe is the drug in humans?
- What are the side effects?
- What is the optimal dose to be carried forward into a Phase 2 or Phase 3 trial?
- Is there a signal based on the Phase 1 data that the drug is both safe *and* effective for a subset of cancer patients?
- Offered to a limited number of patients, often less than 100.

These questions are answered through a process called titration, where clinicians start with a safe dose in a few patients and then ramp up the dose gradually. Each step of the way, the prior set of patients, called a cohort, is thoroughly evaluated with physical examinations, blood studies, and X-rays to determine safety. If a group of participating physicians determines it to be safe, then the next cohort is dosed at a higher level.

But even at this writing, the definition of a Phase 1 trial has expanded depending on the drug being tested. Doctors are designing Phase 1 trials that will tell them if the drug is too toxic and will define the correct dose for Phase 2 trials. In some cases, they expect to see some patients cured even before they have done Phase 3 trials. This is an exhilarating time for patients.

Sometimes, even with continuous monitoring, the drug may prove to be too toxic, and the trial must be stopped for the safety of patients. In my career, I've had multiple studies that have failed either because it was not safe to continue or the drug was ineffective. Patients make a tremendous sacrifice to participate in these trials, and doctors and the industry are very grateful for the sacrifices patients make to make new drugs possible.

Next comes Phase 2, which is only done when investigators have agreed on a dose to be further tested in a larger number of patients. There are two main reasons to do a Phase 2 trial. The first is to further test the drug for safety in a larger group of patients. The second is to determine if the drug is effective in shrinking tumors in the patients tested. To emphasize patient safety is always the first concern, and even after Phase 1, investigators may not know all the side effects a new drug may have. Patients still need to be closely examined by the doctor and have other tests to monitor blood counts. Chest X-rays and CT scans need to be done to monitor safety.

The investigators also want to know how effective the drug is for specific cancers. If the drug shows promise in shrinking colon cancer, then it may only be given to patients with that disease. Rarely do investigators see a 100 percent response for any cancer tested in Phase 2. But a 100 percent response—almost unheard of—was recently reported in a small Phase 2 cancer trial led by the Sloan Kettering Cancer Center in Manhattan. The drug showing this remarkable and surprising response was dostarlimab, a new class of immunotherapy agents for cancer. This is a powerful testimony to the ability of new drugs to have a positive effect on patients with cancer.

Phase 3 studies require hundreds to thousands of participants. One Phase 3 trial may take years to complete and often requires the participation of patients and physicians from around the world. Participating patients are administered the new drug or a drug already approved for the same disease. This is the process called randomization. Patients with cancer participating in a randomized Phase 3 trial aren't given a placebo or sugar pills. Patients with cancer have life-threatening diseases, and it's unethical to offer a placebo as an option. They will always get a treatment for their cancer that is either approved by the US FDA or an effective treatment agreed on by cancer specialists.

I admire our patients' courage because a drug could show promise in Phase 2 but fail to meet the high bar required by the US FDA to be approved. I once led a 300-plus international Phase 3-The Janus 1 trial to investigate a new drug for cancer of the pancreas. Because of the lack of significant progress in treating stage 3 and 4 pancreas cancers, new drugs were needed then—and now. One hundred fifty patients were randomized to Arm A and treated with the new drug. The other 150 were treated with standard-of-care capecitabine in Arm B. When our team reviewed the data with an independent, unbiased team of physicians and statisticians, they concluded that the tumor shrinkage in Arm A was no better than the shrinkage in Arm B. The new drug was a failure. No further patients were enrolled, and we felt there was no choice but to stop or discontinue testing the drug. The study was discontinued.

Martin Luther King marched for Black civil rights. But the whole nation benefitted from his sacrifice. He made us better as a nation—Blacks, Whites, and many others who came after him. When Jackie Robinson broke the color barrier in baseball, it benefitted all. As recent as the 1970s, many Whites believed Blacks weren't intelligent enough to play as quarterbacks in the NFL. Doug Williams of the Washington Redskins

Clinical trials provide excellent medical care.

shredded the favored Denver Broncos to win the Super Bowl in 1988 and proved them wrong. The devastating effects of the Tuskegee experiment were another watershed moment that led to the Belmont Report, which has benefitted all Americans. Since African Americans have given so much to the scientific endeavor, sometimes against their collective will, for the betterment of all, I believe now is your time—your time to take full advantage of the clinical trial protection you have paid so dearly for.

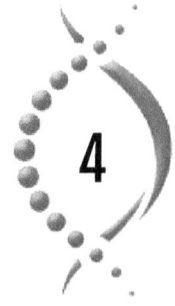

4

NAKED FEAR

"I know the world is bruised and bleeding, and though it is important not to ignore its pain, it is also critical to refuse to succumb to its malevolence. Like failure, chaos contains information that can lead to knowledge—even wisdom."

—Toni Morrison

Simus Michaels is a trim, well-groomed, self-assured Black politician from Southern California, a self-described deist—a believer in God based on reason rather than by revelation. He's intelligent, articulate, and opinionated. He's a local politician and columnist and regularly opines on the African American experience, politics, and the distorted lens through which American history is viewed. Simus is also remarkable in another way. Between 1998 and 2005, he had been diagnosed with two distinct cancers, each in the early stage. Even more impressive, he's now cancer free.

We met by Zoom some months ago, and I wanted him to expound on his cancer journey, including his philosophy of health.

"So Simus," I said, "I've met many patients with a wide variety of views about life and health, and I divide them into two camps. There are the passive ones who avoid the doctor and any thoughts about their health for as long as possible. Then, when a severe illness occurs, they never seem to fully engage in their care. Men are especially vulnerable to this type of behavior. They skip recommended screening procedures, overeat, smoke, and participate in other health-averse activities. These are the ones who are dragged kicking and screaming into emergency rooms and doctor's offices by their girlfriends, wives, or children.

"The other camp knows precisely what their problem is, what diagnostic services should be done, and how their problem should be managed. They have it all figured out. In my opinion, the ideal patient is aware of their body and what the symptoms may suggest, visits their doctors on a scheduled basis, and is informed and prepared to have a conversation with their health care professional.

"How would you describe yourself as a victim of cancer?" I asked.

"I would say I'm somewhere in the middle," Simus replied. "First of all, yes, I've had two cancers, but I don't believe I'm a victim. I was never a smoker, and I didn't drink a lot of alcohol, so by that reasoning, some would say I'm a victim. I reject that. Stuff happens, and when it does, I deal with it.

"Now, mind you, I went for annual checkups. I was very attentive to what my body was telling me at all times. But I was still diagnosed with cancer twice. I love sports, and I like what Wayne Gretzky, the great NHL hockey player, said: 'You have got to skate to where the puck is going to be, not where it is now.' Before I had cancer, I went to the doctor at least twice a year. After I was diagnosed, I pulled out another sports analogy: the doctor is the coach, and I'm the athlete. When I found out I had cancer, I picked the best coach and did exactly what I was told so I could get better. After I got my treatments, I had even more frequent visits with the 'coach,' just so he could give me all the medical tools for the game of life that I needed. I got to do what I got to do."

In the title of his excellent tome on cancer, *The Emperor of All Maladies: A Biography of Cancer*, Siddhartha Mukherjee sums up how most people think about cancer. They may respond to the title in this way: "Cancer is king and emperor of all diseases, therefore all powerful. Everyone shakes in his presence. The emperor is all consuming; he's fearful and demands grudging respect. We hate him, but no one can stand against him."

This has been the case since ancient times. Cancer is the number one health concern of Western societies. Rich and poor, the educated and the dropout, the marginalized and the privileged—cancer is the boogeyman we dread most. So, the dread of cancer isn't unique to African Americans. A UK survey conducted by Charlotte Vrinten found that more than 50 percent listed cancer as their number one health fear. Even more striking, people from ethnic minorities in Britain were more consumed by cancer fear than the White population in the UK.

This has been my observation within my own extended family. Many patients and their families could not bring themselves to even say the word. They would quietly whisper that they or someone in their family had "the Big C." It almost amounted to the evil eye—that which should not be said. A native Liberian American and member of my former church in the DC suburbs

> ... the dread of cancer isn't unique to African Americans.

had been a heavy smoker before quitting some years before she came to America. She developed a chronic cough and visited her primary physician. The doctor ordered chest X-rays and prescribed antibiotics for a preliminary diagnosis of bronchitis. A follow-up visit with her doctor told a different story.

She confided in me as a friend after Sunday Service. "I went to my primary physician again last week," she said as she struggled to suppress a hacking cough, "and the result of my chest X-ray makes me nervous."

"What do you mean?" I asked. "I thought you had bronchitis."

"Well," she said, "I thought I either had TB because I grew up in Liberia or pneumonia. But," she said in a whisper, leaning toward me, "the doctor said it could be, you know . . . C."

I saw the sheer terror in her eyes because even while verbally in denial, deep down, she believed it to be true.

One hot, muggy summer day in Washington, DC, a patient walked into our office for a consultation. She was well dressed, soft spoken, polite, and respectful in speech, as older patients tend to be when coming to see *the doctor*. She had the slight, lilted accent that told me she was from the islands, the English-speaking Caribbean.

She told me the story of her travel to the United States to visit her daughter. Her first grandchild was about to be born, and she wanted to be here in person to welcome the baby. This would be a significant family event that she wouldn't miss for the world. But shortly after arriving in the US, she noticed that many of her dresses were fitting a bit tighter around her belly. At first, she ignored it and thought, *I'm just getting older. Nothing to worry about.* Everywhere she went, it felt like she was dragging around something that continued to weigh her down. She called it a jelly belly. But her dresses got tighter and tighter around the waist. She was increasingly weak, tired, and exhausted by noon. She continued to play down the symptoms but had the nagging sense that something was wrong. The herbal medicines, the rubbing oils, and the bowel cleansers she took were having no effect. When she couldn't stand it anymore, she went to the local emergency room and was referred to a general surgeon, who then sent her to our office for further evaluation.

"Doctor, I can't figure it out. A few months before coming to the States, I went to see my doctor. I thought that since I would be away for a few months, I ought to get a checkup. He told me I was in good shape. 'A clean bill of health,' he said."

I listened to her story and asked some clarifying questions, probing like I was taught to do in medical school. I then examined her but thought to myself, *I've heard this story too many times.* As my examination concluded, I was even more sure that I knew what the problem was, but I kept my counsel until a tissue diagnosis confirmed my suspicions.

An extensive cancer work up was conducted to include CA-125, a blood marker commonly associated with ovarian cancer, CT scan of her chest, abdomen and pelvis, and a diagnostic removal of ascites from her swollen abdomen. The fluid removed form her abdomen yielded cancer cells that strongly suggested she had ovarian cancer. Two weeks later, she came back for a follow-up visit. She was visibly weaker, more tired, and needed to use a wheelchair. I shared the results with her.

"I'm afraid the news is not what you want to hear," I said. "But I have always tried to be honest with my patients."

She began to shake, her eyes widened, and she asked, "How bad is it, Doc?"

I told her that the cytologic studies done on the ascites indicated a high probability of ovarian cancer. She was in shock; you could hear a pin drop. Here she was on the eve of her grandchild's birth, and she had a life-threatening ovarian cancer. It didn't stop there. I told her that based on all the studies, she had an advanced stage and would require surgery and chemotherapy. I told her that the hospital had a weekly Tumor Board, where many of the cancer experts in the hospital gathered to discuss complex cases.

"Would you allow me to present your case at our Tumor Board? We have some of the best oncologists. It is like getting multiple second opinions from these doctors. But when we're done arguing, we'll agree together about how we should go forward to treat your cancer."

"Yes, Doctor," she said, "whatever will keep me alive for this baby."

Our Tumor Board was a lively, high-wire drama attended by medical oncologists, surgeons, gynecologic oncologists, pathologists, radiation oncologists, radiologists, and fellows. The physicians spanned a wide range of age and training backgrounds, some on the verge of retirement who seemed to have seen it all, as well as recent graduates from fellowship programs. Some trained at the National Cancer Institutes, and others trained at multiple medical centers around the country. The case was presented by one of our fellows, followed by radiology results and then the cytology results. An intense debate followed.

"If cytology suggested ovarian cancer, the next steps should be surgery because," one doctor argued, "cytology findings alone aren't definitive to rule out ovarian cancer, and neither does a very high Ca-125. This could be some other cancer. The only way to be sure is to get biopsied material."

"But," argued the gynecologic oncologist, "I don't think she's stable enough for surgery. If I take her to surgery in her condition, she'll probably die on the operating table. It's too risky."

"But the definitive treatment is debulking surgery, wouldn't you agree?" argued another. "Plus, we can get more than cytology. We can get a true biopsy, which will help us know what chemotherapy is best for her."

"No doubt," the gynecologic oncologist replied, "but I repeat, at what cost? The preponderance of data suggests ovarian cancer, and I think the medical oncologist should administer chemotherapy. Stabilize her and get her in better shape, and then I can perform the thorough debulking ovarian cancer surgery."

The hours-long, optimal debulking ovarian cancer surgery was no ordinary procedure. The ovary and uterus had to be removed and multiple biopsies and washings taken; anywhere the visible eye could see cancer, it had to be surgically removed and picked at. Some parts of the intestines might have to be removed if the patient were to have a fighting chance. Only a well-trained gynecologic oncologist could perform this meticulous procedure.

Finally, after raised voices and references to the most recent applicable clinical trial, it was decided. The first step toward optimizing her care ought to be abdominal surgery done by a competent gynecologic oncologist—Dr. Russell Hill, in this case. But she was too unstable for surgery, so the next step would be multiple courses of chemotherapy doublet to reduce the belly full of fluid and get her in optimal condition for gynecologic oncology surgery. Saddened at the turn of events and very much afraid, she agreed to proceed.

She asked me a question, which shook me. "Dr. Dawkins, after all of this, will I be able to see my first grandchild before I die?"

I was moved and still am, even today. But I had to be truthful. That's how I was trained; that was my moral compass. After all, whose life was it? I told her as gently as I could that I could not offer any guarantees; I could not be sure.

I promised that no matter what happened, "You can count on me to do the very best I can for you."

An initial course of cisplatin and cyclophosphamide was administered, and the tumor responded very well. She had the dreaded surgery. She lived—and very well—to see her first grandchild. About two years later, she had her first relapse. She was treated again with the same agents. And again, she responded. She relapsed a second time a few months later, and this time she succumbed. But that fear of missing out on the firstborn of the next generation aroused a fire in her to live, which far surpassed any other harbored fears. She was a winner!

The fear of cancer is universal, and it crosses socioeconomic and educational lines. JT was a vibrant, motivated, and curious African American woman who held a PhD in sociology from a university in the Midwest. Intelligent, engaging, and with a quick wit, she'd relocated to Washington, DC, after graduation to pursue her career. Sometime later, she married a primary care physician.

She was admitted to a hospital suite reserved for the well-connected and the who's-who of the wider Howard University community. She presented with weakness, fatigue, and severe bone pain. Our team was consulted to evaluate her for anemia. Her symptoms suggested that multiple myeloma was a possibility.

Without alarming her, we told her that we needed to do a bone marrow biopsy and aspirate for a more complete evaluation. We examined the cells extracted from her bone marrow under a microscope, and the rest of her labs confirmed our suspicions. When she heard the words *multiple myeloma,* this middle-aged woman, who always seemed to have it all together, burst into tears.

"Years ago, I went to see my primary physician because I was anemic," she said. "After running some tests, she said I needed to follow up with a hematologist because I needed to be evaluated for myeloma. You know, I was a little tired but not feeling terrible."

"So, what happened?" one of my oncology fellows asked.

"Well, I was busy. I received a grant to conduct a research program outside the country, so I ignored the recommendations. I got used to the tiredness. I adjusted to it. The program was going well, so I just kept going."

Now, years later, she was confronted with the reality of her disease that had progressed. Unlike Simus, the columnist and two-time cancer survivor, she had *skated away* from where the hockey puck was expected to be. In fear and denial, she ran away from what she didn't want to hear.

The above examples give two contrasting stories of how different people might react to a cancer diagnosis. One had fear and anxiety but a willingness to fight; the other initially reacted with fright and then flight, with avoidance and denial.

Fear runs deep in all aspects of the cancer journey: screening avoidance, dread at the time of diagnosis, anxieties about treatment effects (hair loss among women tops the list), and trepidation of a relapse, which can be a lifelong concern, often coupled with survivors' guilt.

Many brave and heroic patients have moved from fright to fight and from fear to hope. They've been treated with the best regimen possible. They've been told they are cancer free. But there remains that nagging question—what if? They know, have heard, and are grateful for doctors and the medical team. They're diligent in keeping their doctors' appointments; they eat all the right foods; they pray and meditate. But then, regular checkups can fuel their anxiety. They want to know the results of their last blood PSA as a monitor for prostate cancer or their ovarian cancer blood marker, CA-125. Month after month, quarter after quarter, they hang on to the measurement as if it were life itself. If the values for that visit are low or are trending down, there may be

> **Many brave and heroic patients have moved from fright to fight and from fear to hope.**

a sigh of relief. *Maybe I'll live,* they hope. Suppose lab values are rising without symptoms, or there's a change in CT scan findings even though there's no clinical indication of recurrence. In that case, some will still demand to be treated as soon as possible, even after doctors advise there may not be any reason for concern.

Not far below the surface lurks the fear of death. *What if I should die? What will happen to my family? Who will pay the bills for treatment? Will I leave my children or my spouse strapped with a mountain of debt for years to come?*

> There's another fear that's just as strong. It's the fear related to clinical trials, and it's not unique to African Americans. But within our community, it's a fear born out of distrust.

There's another fear that's just as strong. It's the fear related to clinical trials, and it's not unique to African Americans. But within our community, it is a fear born out of distrust. Even as a Black medical oncologist, at times, I found that this distrust was also extended to me.

Psychological and Spiritual Help

This constellation of fears is well recognized, and some psychotherapists have dedicated their careers to better understanding and treating these fears. Many patients have found that cancer-specific support groups are helpful, and many hospitals offer them as an extension of their services. Some of my patients have shied away from such groups, saying that their diagnosis is way too personal for group sharing, much less discussion.

Simus, the politician from Southern California, believes that it helps some patients to speak one-on-one with cancer survivors like himself, and I agree. He's available to any cancer patient who wants to hear words of encouragement and support. Although science and research drive cancer patient care, hospitals are hiring staff and trained hospital chaplains of various faiths to meet with patients in their time of deep spiritual and existential need to provide health care for the soul, if you will.

Recently, I spoke with a hospital chaplain from Fort Lauderdale, Florida. With more than thirty years of experience and past hospital chaplaincy at Yale-affiliated hospitals, I felt he could give me a real-world perspective on the role of a hospital chaplain.

"Fitzroy," he said, "the role of the hospital chaplain is different from that of a pastor in many respects. It's a *ministry of presence.*"

I wasn't familiar with the term, so I asked him to explain.

"It is," he elaborated, "a ministry of coming alongside each patient and walking through their health journey with them, whatever that journey may be. It's as if you say to them, 'I am here with you for as long as you need me to be.'"

After that conversation, I think most cancer patients could benefit from that ministry of presence, no matter their faith or lack thereof.

5

YOU DIDN'T DO ANYTHING WRONG

"Guilt is always hungry, don't let it consume you."
—Teri Guillements

"We need joy as we need air. We need love as we need water."
—Maya Angelou

G od, sin, and guilt. Three powerful components in the lives of many. Add the ingredient of a cancer diagnosis, and we may get a toxic brew that impacts the way people make decisions about their cancer care and the rest of their lives. In a recent survey of more than 8,000 African Americans and Black immigrants, the Pew Foundation found the following:

- 80 percent pray at least a few times per month.
- 63 percent pray daily.

- 56 percent rely on prayer more than advice from religious leaders when making major life decisions.
- They trust prayer more than their research to make significant decisions. The survey also found that 78 percent believe that prayer can heal.
- 33 percent believe that prayers to ancestors are a source of protection.
- Even among those not affiliated with a religion, 21 percent believe in a higher power.

Faith and religion drive decision-making in all categories for African Americans. For Blacks who are rooted in the Christian tradition, many cling to the Bible verse, "For the wages of sin is death, but the gift of God is eternal life through Christ Jesus." As it relates to cancer, many take the first part of the verse quite literally.

A few years ago, when I was a practicing general oncologist, a patient, Ms. JH, came to see me. She'd been diagnosed with a rare type of uterine cancer. She walked into the examination room, and I instantly recognized her. She was on our hospital staff and was someone I'd come to know very well. She had an excellent bedside manner and was a true healthcare professional. I respected her work. The last time I saw her, she was—as always—friendly, engaging, and competent. Now, she was before me with a healthcare issue all her own. She'd had vaginal bleeding for some time and had been evaluated by a gynecologist, who did a biopsy of the inner lining of her uterus. She was shocked when she heard she had a type of sarcoma of the uterus. Other than a slight decrease in energy, she felt quite well. Cancer was the last diagnosis she expected.

Her cancer was more aggressive and deadly than the more common adenocarcinoma of the uterus. I reviewed the results of the pathology report with her, the radiology findings, and the initial blood work that had already been done. Her referring physician, a colleague of mine, was concerned, and so was I. The preliminary information indicated an advanced tumor. The pathology was a grim prognosis, and the optimal treatment available at the time for this advanced cancer was not very effective.

As I listened to her recount the events that led up to this visit with me, I thought, *There are gaps in her story. Given all the data I have now, the bleeding probably started months ago. She was probably too afraid to have it checked out or thought it would stop by itself.*

"So, Dr. Dawkins," she said, "what do you think I should do? Be honest with me. I can take it. Is there a possibility that chemotherapy won't cure me?"

I had a feeling that she'd already done her homework and had already made up her mind regarding what she was willing to tolerate. These were very appropriate questions from an engaged patient. I knew the prognosis was grim.

"No, it doesn't look good," I told her. "I've not taken care of anyone with this disease before, but I'm concerned. As you know, we have a weekly Tumor Board. I want to get the collective wisdom of the other cancer doctors before making a recommendation. Would you allow me to do that?" I asked.

She knew many of these doctors and had worked very closely with them in her role as an allied health provider, and she agreed. Shortly after leaving my office and before presenting her case to our Tumor Board, she was admitted with complications that included severe pain and heavier bleeding. The Tumor Board supported my initial assessment. No real effective treatment for her type of uterine cancer was available. A clinical trial was her best option. Furthermore, the recommendation from the Tumor Board was that if there were no clinical trials available for endometrial carcinoma, my team should proceed with a doxorubicin-based therapy.

Afterward, I sat with her. Just the two of us sat in her hospital room. I told her about the Tumor Board deliberations and explained that I agreed. I also told her that while the current treatment may not be very effective, clinical trials were always being conducted, and it was essential to hold out hope because advances in cancer research were always a potential lifeline. There was hope. She had no comorbidities and no other major organ diseases that required medications, and the current treatment could at least buy her some time until something better came along. We spent a lot of time discussing her case. There was the potential benefit of a clinical trial at another hospital because there wasn't one at Howard University.

Again, as a health professional, she queried and probed. What were the potential benefits, side effects, and prognosis if she received doxorubicin or participated in a clinical trial? But more importantly, she reflected on her life. She especially wanted to talk about her son. I think he was the only child she had. She talked about how proud she was of him. And how much she loved him and cared about his future as a young Black man. She spoke of some of her regrets in life, things she wasn't proud of, and about God and how she perceived Him. Then, she politely thanked me for the time I'd spent working up, presenting, and discussing her case. But she was unequivocal: She wanted no treatment. I couldn't talk her out of her decision. Nothing I said would dissuade her. Then she rolled over on her right side, faced the wall, curled up in a fetal position, and was finished talking. The sense of finality and hopelessness was palpable.

Had she rejected treatment because of the potential side effects without the promise of a cure, or was it something else? I couldn't be sure. Thinking about it then and even years later, my gut sense after our conversation was that she believed that somehow, cancer was her punishment for some wrong she had committed—and that this was just punishment or a burden she had to bear.

Kate Bowler is an associate professor of American Religious History at Duke University School of Divinity in North Carolina. She was born and raised in a religious community in Canada. Her book *Blessed: A History of the American Prosperity Gospel* was published in 2013. "Put simply," she wrote, "the prosperity gospel is the belief that God grants health and wealth to those with the right kind of faith."

> ... my gut sense after our conversation was that she believed that somehow, cancer was her punishment for some wrong she had committed ...

Put another way, the prosperity gospel is contractual. Strong faith on the sufferer's part obligates God, who is duty-bound, to heal them in the case of a health crisis. Based on the strength of one's faith, if something terrible or undesirable happens to you, strong faith is corrective, no matter what the problem is—even with a cancer diagnosis at any stage. God is expected to make it go away.

It follows then that a lack of cure equals a breach of this contract on the patient's part because God will always uphold His end of the contract or bargain. This was Professor Bowler's belief when, at age thirty-five, she was diagnosed with cancer. According to her, she was prayed for and consoled as would be expected, and the community stood by her.

"But," as she explained to Terri Gross on the NPR show *Fresh Air* a few years ago, "in there somewhere was the hope that I really just needed to find my own spiritual power and harness it and beg God to give me a miracle. And so, there was tons of compassion, a desire to pray for me but also the desire to have me admit that there was something that I could yet do to fix this. And it was hard for me as the recipient of all these spiritual diagnoses to not feel a little bit blamed."

Professor Bowler's story reminded me of the Book of Job in the Bible. Job, the subject of the book, lost his health, children, and worldly possessions due to no fault of his own. But one by one, his three friends who came to console him insisted he *must* be guilty of something. They said, in effect, "Search for and find the sin in your life. Confess it, and you will be restored."

So, there is a layer of guilt because of a lack of faith. Not every religious Black person subscribes to the prosperity gospel as defined by Professor Bowler, but many succumb to that contractual understanding between themself, the cancer they have, and God. *I have sinned; I am unforgivable for something in my past and now have received my just desert. I lack faith, and I'm not healed because I don't trust God enough.*

There's another type of behavior I've seen. I've had extensive conversations with some patients and walked them through a cancer diagnosis, workup, treatment, and the potential outcomes. They listened with respect, patience, and grace. They responded to what I said with a "Yes, doctor" or "Thank you, doctor." But when I ask for their treatment decision, there's a pause, a hesitation, and then, "I want to go home and pray about it first," or some similar comment. That's reasonable if you're a person of faith.

Few of these patients return despite reaching out through telephone calls, certified letters, or known family members. I wonder why they haven't returned. Some probably went for treatment or a second opinion elsewhere. For some, I think there is a sort of guilt by proxy. *If I start treatment, then I don't believe that God can heal me. The only way to prove my faith in God is to avoid treatment, take natural medicines, and wait for a miracle.*

Ms. JH was discharged from the hospital shortly after our conversation. She didn't revisit her decision to forgo treatment, and she died shortly afterward. On the other hand, Professor Bowler, who was very public about her battles with cancer and her views about the Prosperity Gospel, has done remarkably well based on what she's reported through her books and public discourses. She rejected the popular notion of the Prosperity Gospel. She was diagnosed with stage 4 colon cancer at the age of thirty-five and given months to live. As of 2021, based on available public records, she was still alive six years after her initial terminal diagnosis. The American Cancer Society says the five-year survival rate for stage 4 colon cancer is approximately 14 percent. Looks like she beat the odds.

Remarkably, Dr. Bowler reports that part of her cancer journey included an immune-oncology clinical trial after her cancer got worse when the usual treatment she received stopped working. According to public records, this experimental treatment removed visible evidence of cancer. She's gone on to publish another book since the initial cancer diagnosis, *No Cure for Being Human: (And Other Truths I Need to Hear)*.

Remarkable stories, each in their own way. I often think about the ones who never came back after prayer. Did they seek a second opinion? Were they cured through prayer? Were they just afraid and cloaked their fears with the fig leaf of prayer? I may never know.

Faith, according to the book of Hebrews in the Christian Bible, "is the substance of things hoped for, the evidence of things not seen." Faith is personal. For each of us, our belief system is our own, and sometimes, we're clear about what that means for each of us. At times, it's a journey, and we "see through a glass darkly." But whatever our faith or belief system, a cancer diagnosis is a shock to the system. It can trigger irrational behavior. At times, like with Professor Bowler, a cancer diagnosis clears the cobwebs in our brains. It can help us to focus on what's most important to us. Either way, it is a journey, a very personal journey.

As they say, "It takes a village." Cancer treatment and survival require strong and enduring support. So, talk about it.

Cry with others about it. Seek counsel. Seek guidance. On the matter of religion, a pastor or minister of the Gospel can be a tremendous support and point of clarity about what is true and what is rational. Most hospitals now have chaplains trained to discuss such weighty matters as sin, guilt, forgiveness, and death. If you don't have a personal spiritual guide or leader, these hospital chaplains are trained to step into the gap.

> But whatever our faith or belief system, a cancer diagnosis is a shock to the system. It can trigger irrational behavior.

Depression and anxiety are primary mental health disorders among patients diagnosed with cancer. Estimates say that depression is three times more likely in cancer patients than in the general population. These numbers don't tell the whole story, however. Patients create false masks for their families' sake, the treating physician's sake, or their own sake. They often mask their true emotions, which makes it difficult to provide help. The manifestations vary and may be influenced by the stage of disease, type of cancer, level of family support, age of the patient, and the willingness of the medical team to engage with the patient. Screening for depression by health care providers and physicians is not the same from provider to provider, and the availability of appropriate mental health services to address cancer-related mental health issues continues to be a challenge. That said, patients must share their true feelings and anxieties with their treating physicians. Equally, it is critical that their physicians recognize, engage with, and offer the help patients need. Mental health intervention can literally be lifesaving.

Some patients may feel the underlying cause or origin of their specific cancer is due to some personal, moral failing or bad habits. However, the onset of cancer is complex and layered. According to the National Toxicology Program's 14th

Report on Carcinogens, many agents in the environment have a direct cause and effect on the first-time diagnosis of cancer. Sometimes, we breathe in carcinogens, such as smoking and breathing in asbestos, both of which have a high risk of lung cancer. Other factors are all around us, such as excessive exposure to the sun, which increases the risk of melanoma and other skin cancers.

It's important to understand that the cause and progression of cancer are complex. We're still discovering the roots of these disorders. Modern thinking is that there are different types of cancers, but they all have some biological behavior that groups them as cancer. All cancers are a result of genetic disorders, mutations, or distortions that have occurred or are ongoing in the DNA of human cells. These changes are often due to both environmental and inherited disorders.

The origins of a cancer diagnosis may have to do with personal habits and behavior. Smoking, for example, is an established cause of many types of lung cancer, cancer of the head and neck, and bladder cancer, to name a few. However, not all cancers of the lung and cancers of the head and neck are due to smoking. Exposure to radon, a naturally occurring substance that we may not be aware is around us, can cause lung cancer. Certain

> It's important to understand that the cause and progression of cancer are complex. We're still discovering the roots of these disorders.

ethnic groups are predisposed to a particular subtype of lung cancer. The human papillomavirus (HPV) and Epstein-Barr virus (EBV) are two viruses most of us are exposed to at various times. Each one may cause cancer of the cervix or cancer of the head and neck, respectively. Sometimes, we inherit certain genetic risks that predispose us to certain types of cancer. For example, there's a rare syndrome called familial adenomatous polyposis (FAP), an inherited condition with hundreds to thousands of small, noncancerous polyps that grow in the colon. The average age at diagnosis is thirty-four, but can be as young as five and as old as seventy-four. These polyps are first diagnosed with a colonoscopy based on known family history.

Aging, something we have no control over, increases the risk of cancer. There may be many reasons for this, but clinical scientists have found that as we live longer, we're bombarded with environmental toxins that have a cumulative and negative impact on our cells. These lead to mutations or changes in normal cells that may cause uncontrolled growth of these cells. As these cells grow, they continue to change or mutate. They become dominant in the organ system where they started, and they overwhelm the organ of origin. Then they access the bloodstream and lymphatic systems and, like warships, sail away to distant lands to make war in new environments of the body—the liver, the brain, and the bones, among others. So, all of us may regret some bad habits in the past that may contribute to cancer. But it's too simplistic to explain away cancer based on personal habits.

I recall treating a fifty-plus-year-old woman diagnosed with colorectal cancer. She was heartbroken and angry about her diagnosis. She made a point of highlighting her dietary habits when she told me, "I don't eat red meat, so I don't know how I got cancer. I thought that careful attention to what I ate would protect me from cancer."

> ... all of us may regret some bad habits in the past that may contribute to cancer. But it's too simplistic to explain away cancer based on personal habits.

The issues of guilt, if they exist, can be dealt with while also taking full advantage of modern cancer treatments available to fight back. New and effective anti-cancer treatments are developed and are available to the public on a steady basis. In 2022 alone, the US FDA approved more than thirty anti-cancer drugs. Treatment is possible and is increasingly effective. Viewed in this way, issues of guilt become less of a factor, and cancer can be understood and therapy pursued in a more objective light.

There is guilt for some. But joy—yes, *joy*—is a weapon against the tyranny of fear and guilt. And many find it. Margaret Feinberg is a gifted teacher, author, and cancer survivor. She has written extensively before and after her breast cancer diagnosis. In her book *Fight Back with Joy: Celebrate More. Regret Less. Stare Down Your Greatest Fears*, she spills the beans on how she really felt about herself at age thirty-five after her cancer diagnosis and treatment.

She says, "I had anemia, fatigue, rashes, irritable bowel syndrome, mouth sores, itchy eyes, ringing ears, vertigo, chest pain, receding gums, drilling headaches, even nerve pain that felt like electrocution coursing under my skin. They poisoned me until my toenails fell off, and somewhere in there, I experienced an early menopause. There was so much torturous pain."

Even as I write this, I have guilt as an oncologist. I am saddened because, indirectly, it is me and my colleagues she speaks of—my community of medical oncologists. And I'm frustrated that we haven't yet been able to reduce the terrible side effects we sometimes put our patients through. Our treatment has not evolved to the point where patients no longer feel the dread of chemo, no matter what we call the more targeted types of cancer therapies available today. I'm humbled by the courage they demonstrated day in and day out, these patients who subject themselves to what we do. As a doctor, it hurts me to witness what they endure.

Feinberg goes on to say that there were times when she "would rather die." But through it all, she reveals how she found joy. Joy was a self-sustaining force in her life.

Here is how she describes it: "When all the lights go off in life, when everything is stripped away, we can still find a sense of deep shalom in who God is."

There's a lot to unpack in her story. She moved from fear to openness, and she brought her fans and friends on her cancer journey. She certainly was not giddily happy. That was not her definition of joy. Staring into the eye of the cancer storm despite her fears was what it was all about. She admitted the fear but refused to dwell on what might have been. For her, what she could have done or should have done was wasted time and effort. Celebrating the life she had and fighting for the life she wanted for herself and her family was her "salvation." Being in the moment—that was finding joy.

6

HELP! I CAN'T DO THIS

*"There is no time for despair, no place for self-pity,
no need for silence, no room for fear."*

—*Toni Morrison*

The United States is first among equals when it comes to biomedical research, yet within our country, many African Americans don't have access to top-notch cancer care. The playing field is uneven and unbalanced. Joseph Ravenell, writing in the *Journal of the National Medical Association*, said that the lack of access and other barriers are both intrinsic and extrinsic. Intrinsic reasons like fear, medical mistrust, and a lack of health awareness are prominent. Extrinsic reasons include their experience with the medical system and cultural differences. Persistent systemic racism and limited access to quality health insurance or being uninsured are also factors.

A few years ago, a physician colleague of mine recounted a story that took place in his hospital. He was making morning rounds with his team when an angry female patient interrupted them. Three days before, she presented to the emergency department with a high fever, shortness of breath, a severe wet-sounding cough, and yellowish phlegm. A medical workup, including CBC, blood chemistry, and a chest X-ray, confirmed that she had pneumonia. Antibiotics were administered in the emergency room. Then, she was admitted to the general medicine floor.

Bursting into the room, she yelled, "I've been pressing the buzzer for over an hour, calling the nurse for help, and nothing! No one has bothered to see what I needed. Y'all know that I only have Medicaid insurance, and that's why no one seems to care about me. But I have rights, and none of y'all are going to disrespect me! I know my rights, and if I don't get help, I'm going to the hospital administration."

My colleague observed that, on the one hand, she was standing up for her rights. On the other hand, she seemed very defensive because she incorrectly believed she was stigmatized because her health insurance was Medicaid. He explained that no disrespect was intended.

As a result of years of marginalization either due to health insurance challenges, the neighborhoods where they live, or their education level, many Blacks initially presumed they would be disrespected, often based on the realities of other parts of their lives that are carried forward to the health care system. No one wants to feel like or be made to feel like a charity case or that they will get less than optimal care.

Some social scientists who have a passion for understanding and improving the health disparity gap advocate for structural changes within the system. According to the *Black Report* in 1980, published by the Department of Health and Social Security (of the United Kingdom), "Structural intervention attempts to change the social, physical, economic, or political environment that may shape or constrain health behaviors and outcomes." Obamacare was one attempt to take on some of these extrinsic barriers but has had limited success.

More needs to be done if we are to achieve health parity. Unfortunately, many aren't aware of the potential benefits of clinical trials. Others haven't been informed by their physicians. Yet others don't trust what they're being told, and they're potentially denying themselves the better medical care that comes from more frequent doctor visits.

Furthermore, patients who participate in clinical trials are more active in their care, and their chance of stabilizing or being cured increases if they receive the experimental drug. For many, the fact that they may advance cancer care and cancer prevention for the next generation is a motivator.

> **Unfortunately, many aren't aware of the potential benefits of clinical trials.**

The US population has become more diverse. The US FDA, the NCI, and the biotech industry have engaged diverse communities, seeking their thoughts and advice regarding their cancer care and clinical trial needs. These are excellent opportunities to push beyond fears and mistrust and begin to shape a future to be proud of. Americans have always pushed the boundaries, challenging and succeeding where others said we could not. We must win this fight. We owe it to ourselves and our children's future.

What if Jackie Robinson, aka #42, or Doug Williams, the first Black quarterback to win a Super Bowl, had accepted the status quo? Commissioner Bull Connor was the Commissioner of Public Safety for the City of Birmingham, Alabama, an ardent segregationist. This was the same Bull Connor who unleashed water cannons and attack dogs against John Lewis and other marchers as they attempted to cross the Pettus Bridge in a march for Black voting rights. He was quoted as saying,

"There is a city ordinance that forbids mixed athletic events." Robinson knew what he was up against. What if he hadn't helped pay it forward for generations of African Americans who came after him? Doug Williams knew there was a strong belief that the quarterback position was the province of White men. Some even believed that Blacks weren't smart

> What if Jackie Robinson, aka #42, or Doug Williams, the first Black quarterback to win a Super Bowl, had accepted the status quo?

enough to play the position. He rejected that. His staying in the fight has paid big dividends for Russell Wilson, Patrick Mahomes, Dak Prescott, and others. The late Congressman John Lewis, who presented himself as a "stumbling block against injustice," was an integral part of a movement that reshaped the nation's moral compass on civil rights. According to him, he made "good trouble," and his people and all Americans are better for it.

These exceptional historical facts are an inspiration to individual Black patients who are diagnosed with cancer—and their loved ones—to change the narrative from being victims to overcoming warriors. *Inveniam viam aut faciam* (or *I shall find a way or make one*) is the motto of the Holton-Arms School in suburban Washington, DC, where my children were educated for a few years. That motto has always inspired them and me. Be inspired by the past and present heroes.

Barriers, boundaries, and fences—they come in different flavors and forms. Sometimes, they are self-imposed and hold us back from doing what needs to be done, what we know must be done. We can be imprisoned by fear of the unknown, misunderstandings, and an unwillingness to step out of our comfort zones. At other times, the obstacles to better health care are societal or institutional. They're imposed on us and stand in the way of what needs to be done.

Ms. NG was a nineteen-year-old college student at a prestigious university across town. She was intellectual, probing, and confident. She'd earned a full ride to the university and was a first-generation American with roots in West Africa—and the pride and joy of her parents. She went to the emergency department at her university's hospital and presented with a cough and high fever. She was thoroughly evaluated: medical history, physical exam, laboratory studies, and an abnormal chest X-ray. She had a very high white blood cell count, anemia, and a high fever. Taken together, the results suggested a community-acquired pneumonia—or something even more ominous.

By any reasonable medical standards at the time, she needed to be admitted. A more aggressive evaluation was required to get to the bottom of her acute medical issues. But she was not. The emergency department diagnosed her with community-acquired pneumonia. All students at her university were required to have health insurance, which should have given her access to the excellent care available at George Washington University Medical Center.

To her dismay, they wouldn't admit her. Instead, she was told about another hospital across town, Howard University Hospital, that would take good care of her. Even though it was evident that she needed immediate attention, it was clear that someone made the decision not to admit her. This is a practice known as *patient dumping*. Here's how that term is defined in an article by a preeminent medical journal dedicated to Black health issues, *The Journal of the National Medical Association*: "The transfer of a patient from one hospital (typically a private hospital) to a public hospital because of the patient's lack of insurance or an inability to pay."

I later recalled a similar incident as an attending physician. One fine summer day, I got a call from an oncologist about a patient he was evaluating. I remember who it was because he was one of the medical oncologists I'd interacted with as a hematology/oncology fellow. The conversation went like this:

"Hi, Dr. Dawkins, how are you? I have a patient admitted with cancer. I see that you're an attending physician at Howard, and I wonder if I could speak to you about the case?"

I remembered him well, and we exchanged pleasantries about George Washington Medical Center and my days there.

He continued. "My patient is stable but not stable enough to be discharged. My understanding is that Howard University Hospital gets a special subsidy from the federal government to care for indigent patients. Is that right?"

No response. I listened.

"Well, we can't take care of her here, so I'll transfer her to your hospital with you as the medical attending of record."

Except for his brief description of her medical condition—and without medical records—the patient was thrust into our hospital with me as the medical oncologist of record. She was shifted to me because either she had no health insurance or she was underinsured. This was not the first time this happened, and it would not be the last in my years in practice. The doctor left me with no choice because the call wasn't about a courtesy transfer. It was about having a physician's name on record to whom he could offload a patient liability from the private hospital where he practiced.

In many ways, Ms. NG's case was very much like that patient's. She was transferred over her protestation to our emergency department. The workup continued, and she was admitted. After a more extensive evaluation, including a bone marrow biopsy, a spinal tap, and other invasive procedures, she was diagnosed with a rare type of leukemia. The course of treatment would be long, difficult, and high risk. It would require more than one year of treatment if she had any hope for a cure.

She had multiple admissions, an experimental Phase 2 chemotherapy cocktail, and spinal taps with infusions of chemotherapy to clear leukemic cells from her brain. She refused an Ommaya reservoir, a device designed to remove small amounts of fluid from the brain that would also infuse chemotherapy if there were leukemic cells found. She was often in the ICU and had even more visits to the outpatient clinic for chemotherapy.

Our relationship started on a very rocky note. She and her parents questioned my competency as a physician. Moments of palpable anger were directed at me and resistance to the idea that she, a nineteen-year-old in the prime of life, had to be subjected to treatment. In effect, she asked, "Do you know what you're doing?" Her education, a source of pride for her family, was constantly interrupted due to the multiple anti-cancer treatment demands.

On one occasion, when she was in the hospital, she had to be transferred to the ICU again. While in the ICU, we noticed that several of her fingers were darkening and gradually turned black. We consulted our surgical colleagues, who said she had gangrene of the fingers. The only remedy was to amputate the fingers. Our medical team managed patients more conservatively, and we resisted that recommendation. We felt this was a rush to surgical judgment and wasn't a good option at that time. Not at nineteen years of age! We reevaluated the diagnosis and the options. Could it be due to medications? We thought she had a complication from the medications she received. We were in the middle of the classic back and forth between internists and general surgeons, their cut-to-cure versus our conservative approach that would give the body time to heal itself. Over the next two weeks, the situation reversed, and her fingers were saved.

Ultimately, we made peace with each other. She went into remission and continued to receive maintenance therapy, mainly on an outpatient basis. She survived and afterward completed her education. Some years later, she was married and started a family.

The odds were stacked high against her: She had health insurance challenges, a perception that she was just another Black patient without an advocate, and parents who had no experience navigating a medical system that was foreign to them. She had so much to live for, yet so much to dread.

On the other hand, despite her difficult circumstances, Ms. NG had a lot going for her. She was intelligent, asked relevant and insightful questions, and challenged the system at many junctures. She could not afford to lose. Despite her fears, anger, and anxieties, she was 90 percent compliant with the planned course of therapy—not for only weeks or months, but to an oncology management plan that stretched out over years of treatment and follow-up. She found advocates. Her parents were relentlessly supportive. They didn't understand all the medical jargon and all the procedures, but they were committed to doing anything necessary to ensure their child's survival. And she did. She went into remission, and after more intensive therapy, she was cured.

Ms. NG was lucky. Unfortunately, much of health care for the poor and marginalized is based on luck. The system is archaic, intimidating, and even hostile. Reform is needed—in the shape of better access to health care, in patient health care awareness, and patient health literacy. There must be a refresh on patients' understanding and acceptance of clinical trials where needed, not for Blacks but for an American demographic that is expected to be a "majority-minority" by the year 2050.

Patient Advocacy

Patient advocacy is a movement that's taking center stage. Healthcare advocacy is about reforming all aspects of cancer care. Social workers and patient care navigators have been a staple for decades. More recently, small biotech and large pharma are funding clinical trial navigators at individual research sites to walk candidates through the increasingly complex aspects of recruiting and retention. For years, the industry has been under increased pressure from regulatory bodies to ensure that companies who request new drug approval demonstrate a more inclusive and diverse patient population. The need for diversity, the absence of it, and the potential damage to the US social fabric were very evident at the height of COVID-19, given the heated public debate about vaccines, which ethnic groups were at risk, and what we knew about their vulnerability.

There's been a remarkable rise in patient advocacy for cancer patients, and one of the best ways forward is to seek out a social worker at the respective treatment facility. I've worked closely with patient advocates in multiple capacities, including how to move a patient from no coverage to coverage that allows them to receive the care they need. They sometimes seem like miracle workers. They can help the patient apply for Medicaid and Social Security for the underemployed or unemployed. They reach out to organ-specific cancer foundations such as the Leukemia & Lymphoma Society, the Susan G. Komen Breast Cancer Foundation, and the Multiple Myeloma Foundation. These three organizations are well established and have a focus on funding necessary research in their respective areas. But they also provide limited financial assistance to patients. The Cancer Financial Assistance Coalition is a nationwide group focused specifically on the financial needs of patients.

> There's been a remarkable rise in patient advocacy for cancer patients, and one of the best ways forward is to seek out a social worker at the respective treatment facility.

Even patients who have health insurance often complain that they can't afford the co-pays associated with their care.

There is help here as well. One such group that addresses these concerns is the CancerCare Foundation. They manage a list of other foundations and organizations that will help. The American Cancer Society and United Way can also direct patients to additional resources in their local communities.

The system is often overwhelming. Absorbing the shock of a cancer diagnosis can be unbearable. Help in navigating the financial toxicity of treatment is available. Ms. NG fought through and won.

I lived and practiced in the Washington, DC, area for almost two decades. I've heard that many residents' lives are self-contained within the various wards of the city. They shop, go to school, consume entertainment, and go to church in their ward. Except for having to work outside their enclaves, they seem to prefer it that way.

> **Absorbing the shock of a cancer diagnosis can be unbearable. Help in navigating the financial toxicity of treatment is available.**

So, what happens if they must travel outside these wards for their medical care? Who will take them for their chemotherapy or radiation therapy, either daily or weekly? Their children would gladly transport them, but they must work and can't take time off. If the patient is a member of a church or some other religious organization, someone may be able to provide a ride, but it could be inconsistent.

What if they need to get a narcotic prescription for pain? Their local pharmacy may not provide that service. On multiple occasions, I've prescribed narcotics for patients in severe pain who lived in the southeast quadrant of the city. My office is in the northwest quadrant. Because pharmacies were the target of breaking and entering, many pharmacies in the southeast quadrant refused to stock narcotics and made it known publicly. But in the more affluent sections of Tenleytown,

Cleveland Park, and Chevy Chase, there was never an issue with access, so I directed some of my patients there. Still, that was a suboptimal solution because the trip took hours to get from their home to my office to the upper northwest quadrant and back home again in the southeast quadrant. For many, this was nearly impossible. Remember, these were very sick patients. So, leaning on the help of social workers, a social network, church groups, and family can be a lifeline.

One of the remarkable benefits of the COVID-19 pandemic was the increasing use of existing communication technology, such as Zoom and Microsoft Teams, as part of a more significant movement of virtual medicine in clinical practice and clinical trials. Telemedicine has come of age. Patients' visits can be accomplished over this medium on a regular or as-needed basis. You can "visit" with the doctor from your home or office or some other location. Some symptoms can be assessed, and even a limited physical exam can be conducted. In between scheduled treatments, this is a terrific way to reduce transportation demands, cost of care, and undue burden for caregivers, as well as the patients. In other instances, I've overseen trials during the pandemic where arrangements were made to deliver study medication to patients' homes, and healthcare professionals made in-home visits.

Deciding to participate in a clinical trial is stressful for many patients. But if the treating physician with whom a sense of trust is established is also an advocate, then the decision to proceed may be less difficult. In many patients' minds, the treating physician has carefully thought about the patient— their specific circumstances, concurrent health needs, family, work, and the benefits and risks of the proposed trial. There is a basis for trust and a belief that *their* physician will be transparent. The treating physician is *their* advocate. The physician may belong to the same race or social status.

But what if that isn't the case? There are many stories of patients who complain that even when a clinical trial is available where they receive care, available clinical trials aren't offered. Patients often feel a sense of disrespect by physicians in these cases.

Patients may also sense, based on past interaction with the treating oncologist, a feeling they've been disrespected. This may not be the case, but historical events may exacerbate the chip on their shoulder. The fact is, if some doctors think the patient is incapable of understanding complex treatment plans or is likely to be noncompliant with an experimental treatment, they may not take the time to walk through and explain an informed consent form that is often more than twenty pages long. Physicians practicing in an academic center are driven to succeed. They are measured by the number of groundbreaking papers published in prestigious medical journals, the volume of research, and the NIH grants competed for and won. For them, time is of the essence, and if there's a sense that an individual patient is unlikely to participate in a clinical trial, that option may never be presented to the patient.

But many Black patients say they'd like the opportunity to be considered for clinical trials, even if they ultimately reject it. If underrepresented minorities are excluded from consideration, that obviously impacts each study's ability to close the diversity gap that currently exists. Patients also lose the opportunity to get optimal care. Study after study has shown that patients enrolled in clinical trials get better care than those who are not because a clinical trial is essentially a scientific endeavor that seeks answers to a medical unknown. Rigorous attention to the details around potential benefits and risks,

> **But many Black patients say they'd like the opportunity to be considered for clinical trials, even if they ultimately reject it.**

documentation of treatment, and meticulous attention to data collection—followed by analysis—can successfully answer those questions. There's no guaranteed benefit to the individual patient, but to miss an opportunity because they're excluded is a disservice to the patient and the larger community that could also benefit.

Look to the Internet

Access to information about clinical trials through the internet has been a game changer. Patients no longer need to depend on their doctor or healthcare provider to learn about cancer treatment options and clinical trials. Even if patients don't know how to use the internet, their families or communities can help. Children and grandchildren are a tremendous resource. Unfortunately, cancer is still *the dreaded* disease, the one that people of a certain generation refuse to discuss within the family. But the internet is a knowledge equalizer. On sites like the NCI's cancer.gov and ClinicalTrials.gov, you can access free objective cancer information, like the cancer stage, the standard of care for hundreds of cancers, and clinical trials. You can also find support groups, patient advocacy groups, and local and national government resources that can help on a patient's cancer journey.

Choosing to participate in a clinical study may raise new challenges, such as study-related out-of-pocket expenses for doctor visits, lab tests, and radiologic evaluations. Not to mention time lost away from work, transportation to the healthcare facility, and childcare. These expenses may be covered if the study is done on behalf of a biotech company or a government-funded agency such as NORP. The sponsor assumes the cost of the study and all related procedures and drugs, radiologic studies, blood collections, or other activities directly related to the study.

Even so, there could be unanticipated costs. This is a significant concern for the forty-two million people eligible for Medicaid. In January 2022, through an act of Congress known as the CLINICAL TREATMENT Act, all states and territories are required to cover the cost of routine care to all Medicaid patients who enroll in a qualifying clinical trial, which places underserved, marginalized, and disenfranchised patients on the same footing as the insured. The Act won't solve all the problems, but it's another way that advocacy has helped reduce the health disparity gap. Regarding time away from work and transportation, in some studies, patients may receive compensation. But note that *patients are not paid for participation.* This reduces the risk of "professional patients" who may participate in return for money. And finally, if a participant is directly harmed because of the medication or procedure sponsored by a drug company, that company is duty-bound to cover the cost of care, which you can often find on the informed consent form.

STAND UP FOR YOUR RIGHTS

"Of all the forms of inequality, injustice in health
is the most shocking and inhumane."

—Dr. Martin Luther King, Jr.

A thirty-five-year-old woman, dressed in traditional garb that indicated she was of Southeast Asian descent, was referred to us by a gastroenterologist on our teaching staff. At first, we were puzzled because she had no documentation to warrant a cancer diagnosis. She'd arrived in the US about two years earlier to pursue a PhD in physics at a local university. She was married, her husband had a successful career in sales, and they had no children.

She told us about a missed diagnosis, which was every physician's worst nightmare. She had an acute episode of abdominal pain one night, so severe that she went to the local emergency room. After the usual procedures required to check in—a prolonged wait and repeatedly asking when a physician would see her so she could get some relief for the pain—she was ushered into an examining room. After telling the doctor her symptoms and the abdominal X-rays and laboratory studies he ordered were completed, the emergency room doctor reappeared.

"What's wrong, Doctor?" she asked, still in severe pain.

"I think you have peptic ulcers," he said. "I'll write an order for a treatment now and a prescription to be filled at your local pharmacy. Please be sure to see your primary physician."

"But," she countered, "Are you sure? Back in my country, my older sister died of ovarian cancer at thirty-two years old. I remember she had some of the same symptoms I have now. She had to go to Thailand for cancer care. She got better for a while, but the cancer came back, and she died. I'm worried that will be my fate as well."

She did as the physician instructed but had no significant relief.

Again, she went to the emergency room, this time across town. The outcome and the diagnosis were the same. Again, she repeated her family history of early-onset ovarian cancer in her sister. And again, the remedy for peptic ulcers was prescribed.

On a third occasion, she visited another ED. This time the ED at Howard University Hospital. The initial assessment was the same, but she was also referred to my gastroenterologist colleague. After their first consultation, I spoke with him.

"Dr. Dawkins," he said, addressing me in the formal way many faculty and staff address each other, even today, "As a gastroenterologist, I don't think she has stomach ulcers. I'll do an endoscopy just to be sure, but I think we need to do an ultrasound of her abdomen. I'm impressed with the family history she's told the other ED doctors."

An abdominal ultrasound was ordered. A preliminary diagnosis of ovarian cancer was suspected. She was referred to our gynecologic oncologist for a preliminary assessment. After optimal ovarian cancer surgery, she was sent back to our division for management of stage 3 ovarian cancer. She was treated with multiple courses of two drug cocktails—cisplatinum and Cytoxan.

As expected, the side effects from the combination therapy were severe. She had many episodes of nausea and vomiting, complaints of abdominal pain, cisplatin-induced severe pain in her fingers and toes, and frequent after-hours calls with a myriad of other medically related complaints.

All her side effects resolved over time, and she completed her course of studies and received her PhD. Happily, she's still alive more than twenty years later. She's lucky that she's had such a remarkable run, given the fact that she had stage 3 ovarian cancer, which speaks to the power of clinical research to impact patients' lives for good. While my patient did not contribute to the clinical trial that led to the excellent outcome she enjoyed, the volunteerism and goodwill of others directly impacted her survival.

Her knowledge of her sister's history, her sister's age at the time of ovarian cancer diagnosis, the disease stage, the type of therapy received, and her awareness of her risk was impressive. Armed with this knowledge, she didn't settle for a diagnosis of stomach ulcers. Her awareness led her to a correct diagnosis, as unpleasant and unwelcome as it turned out to be.

Family members must share their health journey. You should also know the medical histories of parents, aunts, uncles, and grandparents. This knowledge could lead to early screening or other measures if there's a high genetic risk for breast cancer, as one example. Sharing this information often takes an act of will because, in my experience, we tend to avoid unpleasant and painful stories at family gatherings.

My older daughter had a recent visit to her primary care physician. Before the visit, she texted my wife and me to request written documentation of our medical history. We had verbally shared some of these health facts with her in the past, but this time, she wanted to have a permanent record, not only of our personal medical history but also of our parents.

My other child is equally detailed and perhaps even more assertive about her health care and health needs. Before every doctor visit, she arms herself with the latest information about her health status. She checks with me to determine what additional questions (and often, there are many) should be asked. If a medication is prescribed, she searches the internet for added information, and she checks in with my wife, a clinical pharmacist, for guidance. It seems for her, nothing about her health care is left to chance.

And my wife's mother apprises her regularly regarding family members and their health status. In my Southeast Asian patient's case, she may have saved her life by knowing her family's medical history.

Remarkably, it was only a few years before that the results of a Phase 3 clinical trial published in the *New England Journal of Medicine* showed that with the appropriate surgery, ovarian cancer patients treated with this combination regimen had a much better outcome compared to what was considered the standard of care at the time. Clinical research is one of the principal means by which we can advance medical care and improve the healthcare disparity.

Howard University Hospital is a teaching hospital and is focused on training the next generation of healthcare providers. In fact, Howard and Meharry medical schools are responsible for most of the African American physicians trained in the US. But beyond the teaching of the next generation, I

> Clinical research is one of the principal means by which we can advance medical care and improve the healthcare disparity.

was committed to educating each patient about their specific disease—the complications and the potential therapies—following my mother's legacy as the district nurse. I walked them through multiple serial X-rays, CT scans, and PET scan results so that patients and their families would be more willing to partner in their care.

Often, when I was met with skepticism regarding my proposed plan of care, I encouraged patients to seek a second opinion, preferably outside our institution, which was a trust-building exercise. Many returned more comfortable with my recommended treatment plan. But some didn't, which was their right. There are other excellent hospitals in the area, like George Washington University and Georgetown University-Lombardi Cancer Center, as well as Johns Hopkins Hospital in Baltimore, which is not very far away.

I encouraged family participation. I pointed them to a National Cancer Institute website where they could independently verify the information and recommendations that I shared with them. I was committed to and had a strong belief in the benefits of the patient-doctor partnership. As a teaching physician, it was essential to pass on this vital principle to medical students, residents, and fellows. Caring for patients was a sacred oath, symbolized by the White Coat ceremony, the induction into the medical profession.

This was my opportunity to come alongside each patient, enter their health struggle, accurately assess the issues, and then provide solutions. As a believer in Jesus Christ from a young age, I believe that working out my faith in this way was indeed a calling, not just a job. The fact that a cancer diagnosis often means hand-to-hand combat between life and death fueled my drive to find solutions and provide better care. I embrace the "Conquer Cancer" motto, made famous some years ago.

The results of a recent survey of 424 female patients' attitude toward clinical trials was shared with the American Society of Clinical Oncology in 2022. Of the 424 women, 25 percent were Black. The findings among these 106 Black patients: 90 percent trusted their cancer providers; 83 percent would consider a clinical trial as a treatment option, but 40 percent say they were never told about clinical trials, and even if they were skeptical about a particular trial, they would have valued the information. Why were 40 percent of the Black patients in the survey uninformed? The article didn't say. However, such findings have been documented in other places and by other patients.

Had the survey dug a little deeper, I suspect participants would say they believe the investigators lacked respect for them as potential research candidates. The song "Respect" by the late Queen of Soul, Aretha Franklin, demanded, *Find out what it means to me.* I like the definition found in the Britannica Dictionary: "a feeling or understanding that someone or something is important, serious, etc., and should be treated in an appropriate way."

It's critical to find doctors who respect you as a human being, regardless of your educational level, social status, or economic means. Respect is crucial in all societies, but African Americans are particularly sensitive to and chafe at anything that suggests a lack of respect.

I once admitted a middle-aged Black woman to the hospital who'd been diagnosed with blood cancer. She was engaging and friendly but frightened. It was clear that she didn't grasp the details of what needed to be done and why. The next day, while on morning rounds, I walked in to speak with her. At her bedside was someone I hadn't seen before. My patient introduced the visitor as a friend. She'd been the nanny for his children some years before. He stood up and introduced himself as a PhD in one of the sciences. My patient made it very clear that he was there to help her navigate the complexities of her diagnosis and the planned treatment. He was to be her advocate. I respected the fact that he was there.

The patients' autonomy and respect for their input about their health decisions is becoming more of a shared experience. Conducting any clinical trial is arduous work for the investigator and team. It's both daunting and time consuming to explain in layperson's terms the complex concept regarding how a drug works, not to mention walking patients through a twenty to thirty-page ICF, including side effects and potential corrective actions.

One inherent bias may be to withhold clinical trial options from African Americans because there's a belief that they'll reject the trial or won't understand. An informed and assertive patient shouldn't wait to be asked but should ask about available trials. Such questions may change the researcher's mind to be open to a patient who wants the opportunity to participate.

Help is everywhere if you want to find it—help to better understand what you've been told about your cancer and the proposed treatment, help to get to and from an office visit, and help to formulate essential questions you need to ask when you get to the office.

As Bob Marley says, each patient must "Get up, stand up, and don't give up the fight." I agree. Each patient is their own best advocate.

8

NO LONGER A KILLER; A CHRONIC DISEASE

"What does not kill me makes me stronger."
—**Friedrich Nietzsche**

There's a sea change taking place in the detection, diagnosis, and treatment of cancer. The advances in childhood leukemia have been a resounding success for decades now. I recall meeting a young African American first-year medical student who was around twenty-four years of age at the time. He was smart, worked hard, was soft-spoken, and very articulate. After getting to know him a little better, I learned that he'd been diagnosed with acute lymphocytic leukemia as a child. I understood from my training as an oncologist/hematologist that he must have endured multiple courses of chemotherapy, multiple spinal taps, and intrathecal chemotherapy. Fortunately, he didn't need a stem cell transplant. He went into remission in the early years.

When we met some fifteen to twenty years later, he was cured. A success! Today, we know from the National Cancer Institute that about 98 percent of children diagnosed with acute lymphocytic leukemia (ALL) achieve remission; 85 percent of patients between one and eighteen years old will have a prolonged, disease-free survival, and over 90 percent will survive five years or more.

This success didn't come easy. Multiple clinical trials were conducted, with many mothers taking the risk of exposing their babies to experimental drugs and watching their children undergoing extensive testing. At times, painful procedures such as spinal taps were necessary and were so excruciating that some moms couldn't bear to be in the room while the treatments were administered. These were the brave ones. The courageous ones. The ones who saw a brighter day for their children. They blazed a trail for other children and their parents to follow. They were afraid, but they persisted in hope. The success of treating childhood leukemia is being duplicated with respect to other cancers.

> We've started to think of cancer as a chronic disease—as a disease or series of diseases that can be contained through serial treatment.

Over the last twenty years or so, there's been a philosophical shift in the way many oncologists think about cancer. We now have cautious hope, and we think of converting a nasty, life-altering disease into a manageable one over the long haul. We've started to think of cancer as a chronic disease—as a disease or series of diseases that can be contained through serial treatment.

When and if one regimen failed, new agents would be tested through new drug development or experimental therapy and clinical trials. Cancer was no longer necessarily a terminal disease but one that could be managed, not unlike hypertension. According to the American Cancer Society, cancer is a:

> Chronic disease when the cancer can be controlled with treatment, becomes stable, or reaches remission. Often, when cancer is considered chronic, it will move from remission to recurrence and progression and back to remission. Cancer then becomes a chronic condition that can be controlled with treatment. These treatments may include surgery, chemotherapy, or radiation and are decided between patient and healthcare provider.

What isn't mentioned in this statement is the role of immune-oncology therapy. This therapy has come of age and is a significant addition to cancer medicines, equipment, and techniques. It's a treatment option I'll discuss later.

What's important about understanding cancer as a chronic disease is that patients *can* and *are* living longer, even if the disease isn't cured. Much has been written about cancer survivorship and how these patients can manage their disease and live with cancer while optimizing their quality of life.

Mrs. TG, for example, had an excellent quality of life for about two or three years after her initial diagnosis of advanced ovarian cancer tracking. She *lived* well in between recurrent episodes of cancer. This knowledge, perspective, and positive outlook on life provide context for hope over fear and possibilities over despair. These advances are only made possible through the sacrifice and commitment of brave and forward-thinking patients who, though at times very afraid, push through these worries for their betterment and that of our society.

9

COVID-19

"This person who looks like you has been working on this for several years, and I also wanted it to be visible because I wanted people to understand that I stood by the work that I'd done for so long as well. . ."

—Kizzmekia "Kizzie" Corbett, PhD

A famous comedian on the long-running NBC show *Saturday Night Live* had a few thoughts about COVID-19 and the vaccine at the peak of the epidemic. It mirrored that of some African Americans. He wisecracked, "I've got mixed feelings about the vaccine. On the one hand, I'm Black, so naturally, I don't trust it. But on the other hand, I'm on a White TV show, so I might actually get the real one."

This was brilliant humor, dripping with sarcasm and anti-racist cynicism. Yet, in only a few words, he summed up the dilemma and mistrust of the federal government's narrative and that of the pharmaceutical industry. It was a pervasive attitude in the community across the Black American spectrum. It was also an expression that reflected a shared past and how that past shaped the emerging Black narrative about COVID-19.

Some of my relatives still living in Jamaica often say, "When America catches a cold, Jamaica gets pneumonia," referring to any economic downturn in the States and the consequential impact it has on the tourism industry there. COVID-19 was no ordinary "cold," and by the time the World Health Organization (WHO) declared it a pandemic in 2020, countless numbers had already died, with epicenters in China, the US, the UK, and the EU. It became apparent in the early days of the pandemic that the people most impacted were Blacks and other people of color.

This was centuries-old history repeating itself, this time against the backdrop of another deadly disease. As in the Jamaica example above, while all communities were impacted, COVID-19 had a devastating effect on African Americans and minorities living in crowded housing conditions with multigenerational families under the same roof. Furthermore, due to the nature of their employment, close contact with the public was almost inescapable: public transportation, the food service industry, and providing health care for those infected, to name a few. There was no possibility of working from home or working remotely for them.

These social challenges were heightened by the troubling COVID-19 misinformation that was rampant nationally and nestled in many Black communities. There was talk of Black people being immune to the virus; therefore, precautions against infection weren't necessary. Others posited in the early days that COVID-19 was a hoax. It seemed like everyone had an opinion about the origins of the disease and the warp speed with which the vaccine was being developed.

The mRNA conspiracy theories and the COVID-19 vaccine had a damning effect. The misunderstanding of mRNA's relevance to the vaccine had an explosively negative impact, which led to even greater vaccine hesitancy in many communities, including the African American community. In a paper entitled "COVID-19 Vaccine and Conspiracy Theories: The Need for Cognitive Inoculation Against Misinformation to Improve Vaccine Adherence," Md Saiful Islam and colleagues examined COVID-19 misinformation with data garnered from various online platforms. Among their findings were the following beliefs: "Microchips (nano-chips) will also be introduced into the human body, then 5G networks will enter the business, through which the world elite will send various signals to the chips, thereby controlling humanity," and "The BBC published a travel piece stating that there will be microchips in the future vaccines funded by Bill Gates so they can track who has been vaccinated for coronavirus." Islam and others also reported that some were convinced that the mRNA-based vaccine would genetically alter our DNA, making us different human beings. The suspicions and concerns were endless. In the end, these misgivings by many in the public caught many in the scientific community by surprise. Scientists and physicians were focused on understanding the ticking time bomb they were handed and how to manage and treat it. In this existential crisis, the information void had to be filled. Social media was the forum used to fill that void. Pseudoscience ran amuck.

When it became clear that COVID-19 was no hoax and that everyone was at risk, the avalanche of death was already upon us. It gained speed and became more deadly by the day.

Many who had means left the city in droves. They shifted to hideaways where they could work remotely and in relative safety. They were still able to make a good living and left the risk associated with the food supply chain to others. Some bought or rented homes in sparsely populated mountain retreats. Others flew private jets to New Zealand or remote islands far away from the crowds. Those who couldn't leave fended for themselves against an invisible but ubiquitous enemy.

COVID-19 reeked devastation in the African American community through death by pneumonia. But it was also a harbinger of a "social pneumonia" in the community, the life-threatening pneumonia of mistrusting the system.

The time between December 2019, when the first cluster of viral pneumonia cases was reported by WHO offices in China, to the sequencing of the coronavirus genome in January 2020 was only two weeks. By March 2020, WHO declared COVID-19 a pandemic. The first clusters of a pneumonia (with at the time an unknown cause) but that would ultimately be named the SARS-CoV-2 virus, was first reported in the city of Wuhan, China in December 2019. By March 2020, the CDC declared SARS-CoV-2 infection a world wide pandemic. According to the CDC in March 2020, Moderna Therapeutics began the first human vaccine trials. A mere four months later, Pfizer began their first human vaccine trial, and by January 2021, they had enrolled an astounding 46,000 patients to their trial. At the end of these trials, both companies reported 90 percent better efficacy results.

In the meantime, patients died at an exponential rate. We know now that the tremendous toll was borne by patients trapped in nursing homes, people who were cloistered in unsafe and poorly ventilated living and working conditions, and the poor and traditionally marginalized.

What happened in those first ten months and since was a national disaster and embarrassment. The federal government was caught flat-footed and couldn't get ahead of a pandemic that was predicted to come. Arrive it did, almost 100 years since the last great pandemic, the Spanish flu. This was made clear based on the mixed messages regarding the need for and benefits of masks. So much was outsourced to China that we couldn't help ourselves as a nation. The national economy was in free fall. Our Federal Government was receiving and issuing conflicting recommendations regarding how best to proceed and manage in the face of this unprecedented infection onslaught. Leadership was lacking. Initially, it seemed that the nation was left to care for itself. Americans were caught in the crosshairs of a national political campaign, and like everyone else, African Americans were not spared.

Two other significant factors were particularly troubling as they related to the African American community. A persistent, lingering suspicion of clinical trials—especially in the setting of significant misinformation and fear of the virus itself—as well as the political mudslinging between both major political parties. The White House was occupied by a Republican President whom many Blacks saw as a card-carrying racist. He was brash, crude, and self-centered—a president who spun any national story to his advantage, no matter how disastrous. A circus barker, some would say, for whom the truth was an inconvenience if it didn't serve his purposes.

On the one hand, he presented himself as the warrior-president who was responsible for the lightning advances made in the first COVID-19 vaccines. Yet, on the other hand, he questioned the benefit of the very therapy and the medical experts who recommended we all wear face masks. He was the champion of the COVID-19 vaccine but seemed to suggest that taking the vaccine and wearing a face mask were signs of weakness. By his very example of holding large political rallies at the height of the pandemic while maskless, he may have been indirectly responsible for the death of many of his followers. The year 2020 was the eve of the next national election, and his main goal was to secure a second term by any means necessary.

On the flip side, in the overheated election season, the Democratic party was determined to win back the White House at all costs. Anything that would discredit President Trump seemed to be fair game. On balance, the Democrats, in their zeal to recapture the White House, were not exemplary in their leadership. They played to their large African American base by raising doubt about the vaccine and whether persons should trust the final product. If these were our leaders, what should we believe? Who should we turn to for answers?

In a feverish attempt to discredit the President, the Democrats also played to their base. The result was that many Blacks, caught between their inherent mistrust of clinical trials, a frank hatred of a dissembling Republican president, and a mixed message about the vaccine, either rejected a lifesaving vaccine or chose a wait-and-see attitude.

When the national elections were over, the White House, the House of Representatives, and a 50/50 split in the US Senate, the Democratic leadership declared themselves champions of the COVID-19 vaccine. It seemed all was now well that we had a vaccine that was developed under a prior administration. *You can trust us now* seemed to be their message. We may never know how many lives were lost due to political jousting.

Others have argued that the issue in the African American community isn't vaccine hesitance. Instead, it's an issue of vaccine access. Some national news media outlets made a similar point. In a *60 Minutes* documentary, Leslie Stahl and CBS investigated Black access to the vaccine in Florida under the leadership of another Republican, Governor Ron DeSantis. The piece suggested that many Blacks could only be vaccinated if they traveled inconvenient distances outside their neighborhoods. On the other hand, the well-heeled and the politically connected had great ease of access.

On the contrary, the Black participation in vaccine-related *clinical trials* clearly pointed to vaccine hesitance. According to the 2020 Census, African Americans are 12.4 percent of the US population. Yet in a review of three separate published trials, which was summarized in a review paper by Lana Khalil, Black participation ranged from 3 percent to 9 percent, in the Moderna trials 0 percent to 3 percent, and in published Sanofi trials, a dismal 6 percent. Countless lives have been lost as a result. How will African Americans respond to a new pandemic the next time? Will African Americans embrace the ongoing research efforts to vaccinate against the respiratory syncytial recently approved by the FDA and other vaccines on the horizon?

What's concerning is that the same hesitancy I observed in practice against clinical trials in cancer treatment and a distrust among specific subsets of patients against modern cancer therapy persists. While there were more pointed reasons for the distrust as it relates to the COVID-19 vaccine, that distrust needs to be addressed if African Americans as a whole are to find solutions to their specific cancer-related diseases. Ethical and compassionate clinical trials need to be embraced by the community.

10

JOIN THE FIGHT

"Genomic testing is the future of cancer treatment."

—*Dr. Shayma Kazmi*

"Genes are like the story, and DNA is the language that the story is written in."

—*Sam Kean*

I was chatting with a friend of mine a few days ago. We often meet and compare notes about our families. He's a tall Nigerian American who immigrated to the US over twenty-five years ago to earn his PhD in engineering from Cornell University. He's about fifteen years my junior and still speaks with a very recognizable accent. My wife and I are the parents of two millennials, both girls. He, on the other hand, has three kids. The oldest, a boy, followed his dad's footsteps with plans to become an engineer, and the other two are twin girls. We talked for a while about the boy, who's a junior in college. Then, we turned our attention to our daughters, always a favorite topic of mine.

"So, Fitzroy, how are your kids?" he asked.

"They are doing very well. The youngest is flying back from the Middle East today."

"What was she doing there?" he asked.

"Well, it was a combined trip. First, she spent some time in Jordan on vacation, riding camels and visiting ancient sites. The second half was a graduate school class assignment. She spent time in Tel Aviv to learn about the start-up and innovation culture and prowess of Israel's Silicon Valley. I'm so proud of her and what she's done with her life," I said.

"The other one completed an MBA at Duke's Fuqua Business School and will be flying out shortly to the West Coast for a new job orientation. I'm so excited for her. Both have imbibed many of our values and are now reaping the rewards. The thing that still amazes me, though, is how different they are from each other—like night and day. The other day, I told them about a difficult family situation. The news was not good. As expected, both were sad about what I told them, but the way they expressed that feeling was so different."

My friend said, "That's interesting because I see the same thing with my twin daughters."

"Are they identical?" I asked.

"Yes," he said. "You would think that because they're genetically identical, they'd have the same approach to life situations. But they're so different. It's amazing even to me."

These children have the same set of genes as their parents, as my friend went on to comment, yet they are very different emotionally. One is calm and reserved, and the other is more than happy to share how she feels about any given topic. She's not shy to say what's on her mind.

As I thought about this, I reflected on the similarities and differences in two patients diagnosed with cancer. Their tumor is in the same stage, and they have similar co-morbid conditions (like diabetes and hypertension), the same economic background, and health insurance coverage. And they're both Black. Yet, given the same anti-cancer treatment, one may have mild side effects, and the other may have such severe side effects that the treatment will have to be discontinued. They may have different responses to the same chemotherapy, with one doing very well and the other's disease progressing. We know now that there can be such subtle differences in how one patient metabolizes a drug compared to another based on slight changes in the genes responsible for breaking down the drug after treatment.

The Human Genomic Project was an internationally conceived research project led by the United States. There were two primary goals of the project. The first was to analyze and document all the three billion DNA base pairs in the human body. The second was to identify the thousands of human genes that make up all the cells and tissues in our body and direct how they function. The project would not only provide insights into our oneness as a human species—regardless of race—but it would also tell us how we may be different from each other. Furthermore, success in this task would give greater insights into human genetic variability and how those variations impact diseases such as cancer. Armed with this new knowledge, treatment and medicine could be fitted to suit individual patients with their unique medical needs.

The project was ambitious in scope and began in earnest in 1990, followed by the usual objections about better use of public funds and naysayers opining that the project was bound to fail. By 2003, scientists from the US, Japan, China, the UK, and Europe had succeeded beyond their wildest imagination. Two years ahead of schedule, they had sequenced 85 percent of the human genes. Fundamentally, the project discovered that when we look at individual genes from one human being to another, from one race to another, 99.9 percent of our genetic makeup as human beings is identical. This shouldn't have been a surprise, but we now had scientific proof that we aren't biologically different at all.

But there were some other pleasant scientific surprises, for example, how, as humans, we came to have different traits such as the color of our eyes, the texture of our hair, differences in height, and the color of our skin. As stated by the Human Genome Research Institute, at the gene level, all humans share 99.9 percent of the same genes. The Institute also noted that there were variations within the 99.9 percent of these shared genes, indicating that though the genes were the same, these variations could have profound effects on the diseases some groups may have and their response to medicines.

This begged the question: If the project is all about DNA sequencing and gene mapping, and it points out that we share 99.9 percent of all genes, then what does it tell us about race? Insights into the question of race and what it does or does not mean was never a central question of the project. But it gave us insights and suggested that there's no gaping genetic chasm between the races.

Dr. Georgia Dunston is an African American, a renowned human geneticist, and a graduate of two HBCUs, one of which is Tuskegee University. She received her PhD in Human Genetics from the University of Michigan. She was a faculty member of the Howard University Department of Microbiology and the Graduate Faculty of the Department of Genetics. She's been a leading voice on the science of genetics, race, and implications for human diseases.

In a 2019 conversation reported by *Biologos*, an organization with "the vision of faith and science working hand in hand," she said:

In May 2003, concomitant with completion of the Human Genome Project, the NHGC convened on the campus of Howard University a historic meeting of leading scientists in human population genetics to discuss the significance of knowledge gained from sequencing the human genome to solving problems in society on race. Genetic data presented and discussed at this meeting unequivocally affirmed the biological truth of humanity as one incredibly diverse human race. Evidence-based genomic data show that all humans living today belong to a single species, Homo sapiens. . . The time is now for a new explanatory framework and vision of humankind with different fundamental assumptions about biological relationships defining human identity and population diversity in health and disease. The importance of population variation in the genetic diagnosis, treatment, and management of complex diseases cannot be marginalized or ignored. As medicine responds to these advances by becoming increasingly customized, a more refined definition of both the individual and population is required.

The results of the Human Genomic Project would seem to validate the view of W.E.B. DuBois and many modern-day social scientists that race is a social construct and, in its origins, was an imprecise, ignorant, cruel, and unscientific means of dividing groups of people. That said, some of these apparent slight variations within an individual gene may be clustered together based on geography of origin, such as sickle cell gene mutations predominant in people of sub-Saharan Africa but not exclusively so. Variations of the gene are frequently found in India, the Middle East, and, to a lesser extent, people who self-identified as Italians. We also know that certain groups have clustered behaviors, food preferences, and other environmental factors that may uniquely determine how they respond to some treatments. The impact could be negative, positive, or have no impact at all. This is the case across all races and people groups. At other times, differences in disease outcomes are due to factors such as health disparity based on suboptimal access to health care, the zip code in which some live, and societal marginalization. Some would say that health disparity is the primary driver of differences in health outcomes. Others are not so sure the answer is clear cut.

It's well documented that cancer-related survival is almost universally worse in Blacks compared to their White counterparts. It is also clear that there's deep and variable intra-tissue diversity in one patient, as well as intra-patient diversity of a similar tissue. So, one patient may respond very well to treatment and the other not at all. This is the point Dr. Dunston makes when she says, "As medicine responds to these advances by becoming increasingly customized, a more refined definition of both the individual and population is required."

Medical understanding and the treatment of patients with cancer must become increasingly personalized. Patients should no longer be treated based on old-fashioned racial stereotypes. How best to do this is the basis of government and industry-funded research. To answer this question, more African Americans need to understand the challenge of what's in it for them and see this as an opportunity to help their cause.

In the 1990s, I took care of a Black man with a blood cancer disorder called multiple myeloma. Fully 20 percent of all new cases are diagnosed in African Americans, with a two to three times higher incidence compared to Whites. My patient had just retired after thirty years of work.

> Medical understanding and the treatment of patients with cancer must become increasingly personalized. Patients should no longer be treated based on old-fashioned racial stereotypes.

Now was his time to enjoy life and reap the fruit of his labor. He and his wife celebrated in style by going to Atlantic City to gamble when the city was in its heyday. He was referred to us because of an episode of bone pain while he was at the resort.

As I began my evaluation, he said, "I felt like I owed it to myself to spend some money and begin to have a happy retirement. My wife and I had a great time."

Consistent with my early training as a medical student and internal medicine resident, I allowed him to tell his story, or what is known as the chief complaint and medical history.

"So, why are you here to see me? What happened?" I asked.

I was glad to see that his wife also came to the first visit. I find male patients often leave out important details necessary to round out their version of events.

He went to Atlantic City in a great mood, full of energy and excitement at being able to retire with benefits at age fifty-five from a janitorial job.

"Suddenly and without warning, I began to have this very sharp pain in my left arm." I looked sideways at his wife, and she was nodding in agreement as he told his story. "Tylenol® and Advil® didn't help. I couldn't shake the pain. I never had such severe pain in my life," he went on to explain.

He had no choice, he said, but to visit a local emergency department. "The doctor took some X-rays of my chest and arm. He gave me some stronger pain medications and told me that when I return to DC, I should see my primary doctor."

"Well," I asked, "did the doctor say what was wrong?"

"No," his wife chimed in, "just like my husband said, the doctor gave him some pain medication and told him to see his doctor. But he did give us a copy of the X-rays, and we have them here. We're worried because my husband doesn't complain a lot. You know how these men are, Doc. So, it must be something serious."

"Did he fall or stumble or hurt himself in any way?" I asked.

"No, Doctor. That's what we don't understand," she said.

After completing my review of his medical history and physical examination, I looked at the X-rays using the lightbox in the exam room. I saw osteopenia—really thinned-out bones along his vertebrae, ribs, and upper arms—and it looked like pieces of his cortical bone had been bitten out at multiple spots by rats. A middle-aged Black man: new onset severe, non-traumatized bone pain, and the telltale X-ray findings suggested multiple myeloma. A complete workup confirmed my initial suspicion, and he was diagnosed with that very cancer. We knew even then myeloma had a broad range of behavior, from slow growth with limited symptoms to explosive growth. We also knew in the late 1990s that the treatment options were limited. Velcade, a major therapeutic milestone in treating myeloma, was not yet approved. The average survival after diagnosis was about three years.

Myeloma in African Americans presents about five to ten years earlier than in other ethnic groups. A pre-clinical condition called MGUS, which often progresses to myeloma, is seen more often in Black persons. Frequently, the clinical course is more severe, anemia and hypercalcemia are worse, and survival is shortened. Yet, based on multiple studies such as one done retrospectively with Veteran Administration patients, it seems that when there's equal access to a good standard of care, Blacks seem to do well—if not better—than their counterparts. Confirmation of these results would seem to dramatically speak to healthcare disparity in our system.

Besides disparity, could there be other explanations for the generally reported poor outcomes among Black Americans? Could cancer genetics, the environment, lifestyle, or diet provide further clues? The answers are not very clear yet. However, scientists have found that there may be three genetic mutations found in myeloma cancer cells that may increase the risk in a diverse population of myeloma. Among these mutations (called gene translocation), the frequency seems to be higher in Blacks by about 10 percent. One translocation, in particular, seems to have a better response to treatment compared to the others. Could this be why, when African Americans have equal access to the best treatment, they do just as well as the majority population? The oncology community has not confirmed that. But again, here's another reason for African Americans to help themselves by participating in clinical studies.

One of the substantial advances in myeloma treatment is a bone marrow transplant, which is very costly but has a high degree of success. If a clinical trial isn't available, a bone marrow transplant can be cost-prohibitive for anyone. Even if the patient is potentially eligible, due to the complex nature of a transplant, the inherent risks, and a need for compliance, some physicians may not consider the treatment for Black patients. For the same reasons, some patients may shy away from a transplant.

> What we know about the similarities and differences with respect to cancers like myeloma has come about because some African Americans have stepped up. Many have made sacrifices . . . by participating in clinical trials . . .

Many government and nongovernment funding agencies, such as the Genomic Variation Project, are intent on unraveling this maze of human trait variations, environment, drugs, and social determinants to better understand their role in human diseases. What we know about the similarities and differences with respect to cancers like myeloma has come about because some African Americans have stepped up. Many have made sacrifices by a commitment to their interest and that of their children by participating in clinical trials, have provided cancer tissue for research, or have given consent for their clinical data to be studied so that clinicians and scientists can help move the disparity ball forward. We need more warriors like this.

Over my first fourteen years of practice, I had the privilege of caring for some remarkable patients. Some are more memorable than others because of their grace and grit under overwhelming, heartbreaking circumstances. About five years after completing my fellowship at George Washington University, a young Black woman, less than thirty years old, walked into my exam room. She was referred to me for an initial breast cancer consultation. She was a single mom, either uninsured or insured by Medicaid; I cannot recall now. She lived in the Southeast quadrant of Washington, DC, in one of the poorer and marginalized wards of the city.

She had broken an arm after falling down a flight of stairs and sought initial care in the emergency department of a local hospital in Anacostia. Ms. TM had her medical records and X-rays from her ER visit, which I reviewed with her. The working diagnosis: rule out breast cancer and appropriate assessment since cancer isn't diagnosed until there is a confirmatory tissue biopsy. Remarkably, her report of the events leading to the initial visit was the same one provided to me. According to her, a daily grind of working, caring for her young daughter, and just trying to survive was her routine. On the day she visited the DC General Hospital in her neighborhood, all was well, and she had no health concerns until she slipped on a banana peel, fell, and broke her arm.

I asked her to remove her shirt so I could examine her. When she did, a foul odor filled the room. Her left breast was ulcerated, oozing a pus-like bloody material. Not once during medical history did she speak of the mass in her breast. She seemed oblivious to it. She insisted that the only concern she had was the broken left arm. Yes, the initial bone X-ray clearly highlighted a pathologic fracture. However, I was struck by her focus and am still pained by the power of denial that I thought was evident in Ms. TM. She had a pathologic fracture because of breast cancer that had spread to the left arm.

After a complete workup, including a breast biopsy, blood studies, and CT scans, the pathology report confirmed breast cancer of a very virulent type: triple-negative breast cancer. We know now from years of research that the prevalence of this type is twice as frequent, more virulent, and occurs at a younger age in African and African American women. The overall survival is also shorter. Are these alarming clinical outcomes the results of genetics only, or are they a combination of environmental factors, lack of access, and other health disparities?

The role of fear and denial has a greater impact on cancer outcomes than many may realize. Ms. TM's story, even back in the late 1990s to early 2000s, should have been a rare occurrence. Unfortunately, during my time at the university, she wasn't the only one presenting with far-advanced metastatic cancers of all types. There were other ulcerated breast cancer cases and at least one mummified left breast cancer in a postmenopausal, well-educated, and married African American woman of means. The list was, unfortunately, too long.

> **The role of fear and denial has a greater impact on cancer outcomes than many may realize.**

According to the American Cancer Society, Black women have a lower incidence of breast cancer compared to the majority population. However, the outcomes trend worse compared to the majority population. Like many other cancers, breast cancer has many variants, and some are more benign than others. Others have a well-established and often aggressive genetic profile. Post-menopausal breast cancer tissue with estrogen and progesterone lends itself to treatment with drugs like tamoxifen, and yet others diagnosed in premenopausal women aren't amenable to hormonal therapy.

Dr. Olopade, an African American of Nigerian descent and 2005 recipient of the MacArthur Genius Award and Professor of Medicine at the University of Chicago, has been on the frontlines of uncovering the relationship between race, inherited cancer risks, and narrowing cancer health disparity. Triple-negative breast cancer (TNBC) is one of the most aggressive breast cancer subtypes. It traditionally does not respond well to chemotherapy, estrogen therapy, or some of the more standard therapies administered to women diagnosed with breast cancer. Though, happily, there have been encouraging advances in the field over the last five to ten years.

We know that more Black women are diagnosed with this cancer compared to White women—twice as many, in fact. More Black women present with the disease at an earlier age, have a more advanced stage when first diagnosed, and have a higher death rate or mortality compared to Whites. This fact has been observed both here in the United States as well as in Black women in West Africa. Scientists have known this for some time now. The National Cancer Institute (NCI) is very much aware of this. As a result, there are ongoing investigations to understand why and what can be done about it. One way to further investigate would be to design drugs that attack this type of breast cancer and then study how effective these could be in clinical trials. But the most vulnerable and at-risk women will need to assist in providing answers. My patient was treated with a doxorubicin-based chemotherapy regimen at the time. But because she had metastatic, triple-negative breast cancer at the initial diagnosis, including to her liver and bones, she didn't do well.

Today, much more is known about TNBC, and as of this writing, the US FDA has approved at least five drugs to treat this disease. Alarmingly, only one Phase 3 trial leading to US FDA approval enrolled 10 percent or more Black women. There are multiple reasons to explain these low rates of enrollment. Access and availability in disadvantaged neighborhoods and a lack of awareness are two that come to mind. One of the consistent complaints from Black patients is that they don't have access to these potentially life-saving trials. Or if these trials are being conducted at a center near them, the option isn't offered. We hear from patients that they want to be included and informed, and they understand the benefits of clinical trials and the importance of paying it forward.

Hearing these complaints, I think back to my two daughters when they were no older than five years old. Looking forward to when they would become young women, I worried for them and their risk. The Komen Foundation has been leading the fight to raise breast cancer awareness for decades. The Komen's Race for the Cure was a highlight for our cancer center. One year, I took our two girls in a red wagon, pulling them along for the race around the Washington Monument. These pictures have been used to reinforce the need for better breast health care as they mature.

Conducting a clinical trial is complex, infused with multiple regulatory demands, and time consuming for patients and investigators. Thus, some investigators may calculate that their time is best spent discussing a clinical trial with patients who are more likely to agree. That behavior isn't acceptable. Black patients have said that they're more likely to trust and consent to a clinical trial if members of the team, and especially the investigator, look like us. Diversity in the workforce is critical if we are to see an ongoing improvement in African Americans enrolled in clinical trials. In a report presented by ASCO 2020 Virtual Scientific Program, less than 5 percent of all hematologists and medical oncologists in the US self-identify as Black. Rarer still the percentage focused on clinical trials. That said, Black patients owe it to themselves as healthcare consumers to arm themselves with the relevant information when they go to see their doctor. If not invited to participate in a clinical trial because of historical perceptions, then they should ask. If they ask and are refused before going through the rigorous eligibility criteria, then patients should complain. This is a right as an American.

There is, in my opinion, no further excuse for African Americans to be passive about their health needs. The world of healthcare is changing, and a significant component is self-advocacy and patient advocacy. The status quo is no longer acceptable.

At the height of the George Floyd fiasco, my children asked me in effect: "Dad, what positive impact have you had on race relations in America?" It was a direct question and one laced with frustration. But it was also a blunt challenge to me. Asked another way: "Dad, what kind of America are you leaving behind for us, your kids?" In some ways, I took it as a stinging rebuke.

The drive toward a better understanding of the role of human genetics, the genetics of individual cancers, human variation,

> Participating in and demanding the opportunity to contribute to better health through clinical trials and the scientific process should not be dismissed by African Americans.

the environment, and health disparity is ongoing. Many of the leading African American scientists, clinicians, and thinkers understand these are complex questions without simple answers. But they are questions that need to be asked and scientifically pursued. Regarding human genetic variation, the FDA commissioner repeats an accepted fact when he said:

> It is known that biological differences exist in how people respond to certain therapies. For example, variations in genetic coding can make a treatment more or less toxic for one racial or ethnic group than another. These variations

can also make drugs like antidepressants and blood-pressure medications less effective for certain groups.

Many, like Drs. Olopade and Dunston, as well as others in the Black scientific and clinical research community, understand this. It's probably true that the concept of precision medicine, which proposes that "disease treatment and prevention that takes into account individual variability in genes, environment, and lifestyle" is an excellent way forward, which seeks to predict and not just react to the medical needs of patients as individuals. Participating in and demanding the opportunity to contribute to better health through clinical trials and the scientific process should not be dismissed by African Americans.

ON THE SHOULDERS OF GIANTS

"I can positively state that the Soviet Union will not be beaten by the United States in the race for a human being to go to the moon."

—Vladimir Komarov, Soviet Cosmonaut

"We choose to go to the moon in this decade and do the other things, not because they are easy, but because they are hard." With that, the tanned, photogenic, and charismatic thirty-fifth President of the United States, John Fitzgerald Kennedy, ignited America's race to put the first man on the moon. The Cold War was at its zenith. The enemy, the Soviet Union, had threatened to "bury" us. Kennedy recognized the threat, understood the risks of inaction, and rose to the challenge. His Houston speech at Rice University made that clear.

Kennedy's vision was much larger than victory over the Russians. Landing the first man on the moon would provide opportunities for all humankind. It would be a giant stroke of genius, demonstrating boundless scientific possibilities. On the road to victory, the American moonshot was filled with political drama and arguments, missteps, mishaps, underfunding, and budget overruns. In 1969, some seven years after Kennedy's death, the dream came true when Neil Armstrong said, "The eagle has landed." The United States had done the hard thing. We put the first man on the moon. Those were heady days when we believed, as a nation, that not even the sky was the limit to what was possible.

Fast forward two years later, in 1971, when another president, the infamous Richard Milhouse Nixon, lit a different fuse that would ignite the War on Cancer. It was officially called the National Cancer Act of 1971. The goal was to amend and strengthen the National Cancer Institute to lead the national effort against cancer. The "War on Cancer" was a nice sound bite. Cancer as the enemy was on the move, on the attack; thousands of people died annually, and we, as a nation, were falling back. There didn't seem to be any forward progress. We needed a new direction—a course correction—or else we would be overrun. Indeed, with adequate funding, a revamped strategy, and a can-do spirit, we could first blunt the attack and then make significant advances. Perhaps the fight against cancer could have its moon landing.

To understand how far we've come in the fight, we must understand where we've been. We need to know who some of the primary movers and shakers were. How was the war fought, and what do we have to show for it? As an Act of Congress, the War on Cancer had a powerful and positive impact on the dramatic improvements we see in the research and outcomes of cancer today.

In the early 2000s, a young man walked into my office for a consultation. We exchanged the usual pleasantries that happened between a new patient and a medical consultant. Then we got down to the business of why he came to see me. He was about average height and had the complexion of someone from East Africa. He moved slowly, and it appeared he hadn't had a good night's sleep. Dressed in an open shirt, chinos, and a long white coat with a stethoscope draped around his neck, his attire seemed hastily put together. He was pleasant and spoke in a halting accent, which was consistent with many from that region of Africa.

As we talked, I realized I had seen him before. In fact, he was an internal medicine resident doing his medical rounds at our hospital. Just about all the internal medicine residents would rotate with me at least once over three years. He hadn't. He'd completed medical school and a mandatory one-year internship in his home country, then migrated to America for specialty training. I took his medical history, starting with, "Why are you here to see me?"

Dr. AW said, "I have a high fever. I'm tired all the time. I have no energy, and at night, when I'm on call, it's the worst. When I get home after a thirty-six-hour shift, it's all I can do to crawl into bed. I feel full all the time, even when I have not eaten much food."

I recalled my shifts as a resident, but I experienced nothing quite like what he endured. He was pale and looked drained. His examination was impressive for having an enlarged spleen, the internal abdominal organ typically located below the left side of the diaphragm and protected by the rib cage. In Dr. AW's case, the spleen was so large that I had no difficulty palpating it because it was at least five centimeters extended beyond the lower end of the rib cage. There was danger here because sometimes, with such a large spleen, just the act of a too-aggressive examination could cause it to rupture, and a patient could bleed to death. His enlarged spleen gave me an additional clue to his poor appetite. Not only was it extended below the rib cage, but it could also mean that it extended upward, compressing his stomach. It would only take a small amount of food to cause him to feel full since the stomach couldn't expand to accommodate more food.

I completed the rest of his examination. I reviewed his medical records. He had a very high white blood cell count (WBC), a low hemoglobin and hematocrit, and a reduced platelet count. Completing his daily ward rotation was draining.

"Well, Dr. AW," I said, "based on the limited information I have, it appears that you have a type of leukemia. I don't know which yet, but it doesn't seem to be an acute type because you've had these symptoms for months now."

After a medical workup, as he and I suspected, a diagnosis of chronic myelogenous leukemia (CML) was confirmed. Based on the laboratory data, he had the *sine qua non* of CML, the Philadelphia chromosome, found in over 90 percent of patients with this disease. Leukemia, a type of blood cancer, often triggers fear and worry for patients and their doctors. But in his case, this was chronic leukemia. It was still concerning, but it had a better prognosis than acute leukemia in adults. Without treatment, patients die, but with effective treatment, they could live with the disease for years.

We started him on a standard of care with a drug called interferon. Interferon was administered by subcutaneous injection, and it had been the standard of care for many years. The problem was that it was somewhat helpful at treating CML but also quite debilitating with side effects such as flu-like symptoms, fever, headache, nausea and vomiting, and problems thinking clearly at times. My heart went out to this young doctor because in treating CML, interferon could exacerbate many of the symptoms he had due to the disease. But then, on the other hand, it would help to reduce his WBC, improve anemia, reduce the size of his spleen, and possibly improve his appetite.

He said, "Dr. Dawkins, I'll do whatever it takes. If this is the best that is available, then there's no question I'll do what is necessary. I came to the US to become a medical specialist, and I intend to complete the course no matter what it takes."

We both realized that new, more effective therapy with fewer side effects was needed.

Dr. AH was on this toxic but somewhat effective CML treatment with interferon for a little over one year. I admired his pluck. He was diligent and attentive to the patients under his care. He never complained and was a ray of sunshine whenever I saw him.

Shortly afterward, it happened—a therapeutic breakthrough—what would be a significant milestone in the treatment of CML. There were preliminary reports of a drug called imatinib, which had shown promise. The guinea pig and other animal studies had been done. Exposing humans to the drug would be the next step. The drug safety profile had been completed in Phase 1 trials, and the early promise of a positive effect was observed in Phase 2 studies. Imatinib seemed to hold great promise but was not approved by the US FDA because the ultimate proof of benefit based on Phase 3 trials had not been done. But now, at last, as reported by the premier journal, the *New England Journal of Medicine,* the results of an exciting Phase 3 clinical trial showed the superior benefits of imatinib, also known as Gleevec, for CML sufferers.

Phase 3 clinical trials, confirmed with clear scientific evidence, proved that the drug is effective. Almost 90 percent of the people who got the treatment on one arm of the study responded. But only 37 percent responded on the other. There was excitement in the medical oncology and hematology community. This was so significant that the findings were on the front page of *Time* magazine. Among other things, Gleevec's efficacy resulted in suppression of the Philadelphia chromosome, improved anemia, and reduced WBC and leukemic cells, and an improvement in my patient's stamina, appetite, and feeling of well-being were all documented.

Dr. AW was initiated on Gleevec within weeks of the *NEJM* publication. The turn of events was like a man who lived a nightmarish existence on a daily basis, who then awoke to a burst of hope and the possibility of a new life. His appetite improved. He was less exhausted at the end of his nights on call. His spleen size was reduced, and his spiking fevers went away. He was a rejuvenated resident and plunged into his career with even greater enthusiasm.

About two years into Gleevec therapy, he returned to his home country and got married in a traditional Islamic ceremony. He returned with his bride to Washington, DC, and then had an American-style wedding to which my wife and I were invited. It was a joyous occasion. For the first time, we heard an Ethiopian minstrel brought in for the occasion. He sang for well over an hour, nonstop, to the praises and the beauty of Dr. AW's bride. Such was the custom of East Africa that I hadn't experienced before. I often think back with gratitude to the participants who took the leap by enrolling in the multiple Gleevec trials that made this successful treatment possible and allowed me to see such a happy day for my now-former resident.

Dr. Brian Drucker, a clinician at Oregon Health Science University, led the Gleevec studies and was one of the bright lights that traced its success to funding the National Cancer Institute and Nixon's War on Cancer.

But the War was not happenstance, not simply a by-product of the federal government's foresight. The likes of the Laskers, Mary and Albert, had waged a long national campaign. According to the Mary Lasker Papers, she was a "medical philanthropist, political strategist, and health activist who acted as the catalyst for the rapid growth of the biomedical research enterprise in the United States after World War II.

Called 'a matchmaker between science and society' by Jonas Salk." But who was she, and what made her tick? Upon her death in 1994, the dean of Harvard School of Public Health said in the *New York Times*, "Mrs. Lasker was an extraordinary woman who transformed our nation's capacity for science discovery." She was born and nurtured on the "milk of public service," in Watertown, Wisconsin, in 1900. Her mom was a campaigner for public beautification with flowers, trees, and parks. The young Mary watched, observed, and imbibed her mother's passion for doing good in the service of the public.

But when both her parents died of hypertension-related strokes when Mary was in her thirties, her public service became fueled by anger. She's quoted as saying, "I'm as opposed to heart attacks and cancer and strokes the way I'm opposed to sin."

She was an accomplished businesswoman long before it was acceptable. She campaigned for continued improvement in parks and other public beautification projects, just like her mother. Now, there was the added urgency to take on health care in the public interest. But how could she do this?

She had divorced her first husband ten years earlier when she met and married her second husband, Albert Lasker. Albert was a leader in the advertising business. He had built a very successful advertising agency as an executive at the Lord and Thomas agency in New York. The firm had a national reach. Years before, he was a noteworthy mover in the campaign of President Warren Harding. Harding, in turn, appointed him to the United States Shipping Board, which opened new network avenues for the very ambitious and forward-thinking Lasker.

Self-assured and unwilling to take no for an answer, Mary brought a passion for public service to the marriage but had limited access to power. Albert brought political savvy and wealth. According to the *NIH Profiles in Science*:

The Laskers drew on their money, connections, and high-profile foundation to garner federal financing of medical research, a controversial idea at a time when such research was the domain of universities, non-profit institutes, and private business. They concentrated on cancer, mental health, and birth control and later added heart disease, arthritis, and hypertension. Their first project was to reorganize the American Cancer Society by committing it to large-scale fundraising, publicity, and lobbying campaigns.

Together, they joined forces. He knew the power of advertising to sell an idea and to change minds. She drew on her experience as a businesswoman as she entertained and hosted the powerful, the influential, the mighty—the movers and shakers on the national scene. Intelligent, focused, and relentless, she button-holed members of Congress and senators, cajoled captains of industry, and bent their wills toward her goal.

The cancer death rate was alarming. Knowledge of the true prevalence, the incidence, and how cancer spreads or metastasizes was, at the time, rudimentary at best. Together with scientists and physicians, they concluded that cancer was a national scandal. In 1950, the US population was estimated to be 150 million persons. By some estimates, cancer killed two hundred thousand persons annually.

To change the death-spiraling trajectory, massive funding for clinical research was urgently needed. They understood that the relative pittance allocated for the National Cancer Institute's annual budget would not do. Central to their vision to transform the fight against cancer was a national campaign to raise public and government awareness about cancer. The second goal was to encourage or badger the federal government to adequately increase funds for the NCI and to empower the institute to spearhead the fight. It was a winning combination.

Even after Albert died from colon cancer in the 1950s, she soldiered on through the efforts of the Lasker Foundation. It reflected true American activism in the public interest. But they were not alone in the fight as they waged this relentless campaign against a national scourge.

Physician-scientists from their unique perch sounded the alarm. In laboratories, in operating rooms, in medical societies old and new, there was a rising sense of trepidation. America needed a new strategy to combat this deadly disease. And without proper organization and better funding, we could not defeat this relentless enemy.

Up until the 1970s, cancer diagnosis, management, and treatment were dominated by the "big three" specialties. First, *surgeons* were kings of the hill. For more than a half-century, the Halstead doctrine of breast cancer surgery, for example, held sway. Halsted believed and taught, with very little objective data, that in the surgical management of breast cancer, no matter how small the lesion or large, more was better. Cold steel on warm flesh, aggressively applied, was the answer.

But there was the tiny issue of micrometastasis, small pockets of cancer cells that traveled undetected from the original site to other organs such as the brain, lung, and bone. This was poorly understood or studied at the time. Think about a dandelion plant growing on a bright green, well-manicured lawn. It is fully mature, and only tiny feathery seeds are left. Pulling up the plant by the root is good. But in the process, the many small, tiny seeds float away, out of sight and mind. Spring returns the following year, and with it, not just one lone dandelion but hundreds on the same verdant, green lawn. This is the nature of cancer metastasis. Initially out of sight and unless treated with medications, it often returns with a vengeance unless it is treated before it becomes obvious. Surgery or radiation therapy alone was not the answer. These gaps in our understanding of the nature of micro-metastasis, who is at risk, how it can be detected, and when and how to treat it were medical and scientific gaps that had to be plugged.

The second dominant field was *radiation oncology*, which had its roots in Germany over 125 years ago. It was presented in a paper titled "Concerning a New Kind of Ray" by Wilhelm Conrad Roentgen. These rays were subsequently dubbed X-rays. Closely aligned with the surgical management of cancer, radiation oncology was focused on local management—treating small pockets of localized cancer that weren't removed at the time of surgery. At other times, radiation therapy is used to control cancer that's spread to other anatomical sites or used as palliation to control pain. Yet again, like in surgery, the focus was on the local disease with minimal impact on the microscopic cells that had already hijacked the blood and lymphatic systems and were swimming downstream to other organs such as the liver and kidney.

The third was the study of *pathology*. The focus here was the study of human diseases, their causes, effects, and natural history. In the case of cancer, making a diagnosis was based on obtaining tissue of the diseased area by biopsy or examining leukemic cells under a microscope. Pathology defines the location, the nature of, and the microscopic characteristics of disease. Since then, the study of pathology has rapidly evolved into a mainstay of cancer management.

The big three dominated the field for decades, but that was about to change. The role of the *chemotherapist* as a potential fourth arm of the management of cancer was, until then, very much in its infancy. The chemotherapeutic approach to cancer care was not initially considered a sizable factor that could advance cancer research and treatment. The early agents for treatment were essentially modified chemicals with very toxic side effects. Unfortunately, we've come to know these early treatments as chemotherapy because, even now, many perceive that all chemotherapy is poisonous. Even in the 1940s and

1950s, there were some early successes of these therapies in treating leukemia.

In 1964, seven remarkable physician-scientists, stalwarts in their field, and visionaries founded the American Society for Clinical Oncology (ASCO). But at the time, little attention was paid to these chemotherapists. At best, they were seen as bit players in the management of cancer. Seven medical oncologists focused their cancer research (primary as well as clinical trials) using chemotherapy—six men and one woman.

These seven believed a new approach was needed to conquer cancer, and a society of like-minded thinkers would barnstorm into cancer treatment to create a space that effectively revolutionized cancer care for the better. To be clear, in the early days, some of these people were trained surgeons who began to understand the limitations of surgery, radiation therapy, and pathology research. They felt that issues of distance metastasis, detectable or microscopic, was a fertile field of research. Jane C. Wright, MD, a surgeon by training and one of the pioneers in the field of chemotherapy, was quoted as saying chemotherapy is the "Cinderella of cancer research for its incredible potential in treating multiple types of lethal cancer."

They were Arnoldus Goudsmit, Fred J. Ansfield, Herman A. Freckman, Robert Talley, Harry F. Bisel, William Wilson, and Jane C. Wright. Their very first meeting was at lunchtime in the Edgewater Beach Hotel in Chicago in 1964. A new society was born. Indeed, they wanted to explore, like President Kennedy's vision for moon exploration, the outer limits of what was possible. These new emerging chemicals could be transformational. Like Armstrong and other American moon explorers who came after them, they were pioneers going beyond the bounds of the big three, seeking new therapies to fight a relentless enemy.

Jane C. Wright wasn't just the only woman in this illustrious group; she was a Black woman. She was a surgeon, a clinical scientist, and a pioneer from a dynasty of Black physicians, including her father, Dr. Louis Tompkins Wright, a Harvard-trained physician with whom she performed groundbreaking chemotherapy experiments at Harlem Hospital in Manhattan. Her obituary in the *New York Times* in 2013 described her as "Dr. Jane C. Wright, a pioneering oncologist who helped elevate chemotherapy from a last resort for cancer patients to an often-viable treatment option . . ."

Her backstory is fascinating. Her paternal grandfather, Dr. CK Wright, was born into slavery, and after emancipation, he attended Meharry Medical College, where he graduated as a physician. Her step-grandfather was Dr. William F. Penn, who graduated from Yale University with a medical degree. Her father, Dr. Louis Tompkins Wright, was one of the first African Americans to graduate from Harvard University Medical School. He further distinguished himself while working at Harlem Hospital in Manhattan, when he established the Harlem Cancer Research Foundation. As early as the 1940s, he'd already begun to explore the potential benefits of chemicals that could be used to treat cancer.

> Jane C. Wright wasn't just the only woman in this illustrious group; she was a Black woman. She was a surgeon, a clinical scientist, and a pioneer from a dynasty of Black physicians . . .

Dr. Jane C. Wright graduated from Smith College in Massachusetts and enrolled at New York Medical College in 1945. Her rise as a chemotherapist, soon to be known as a medical oncologist, began when she joined her father in his Harlem Hospital laboratory. She distinguished herself by suggesting that the cancer tissue removed from patients was the best medium for testing various chemotherapeutic agents. The field was in its infancy, and for years after, her approach to matching specific chemotherapeutic agents to specific cancers was considered novel.

In the earlier years of my career, some medical oncologists were still exploring this option, even though, at the time, it was beginning to fall out of favor. Dr. Clifford Hudis, a past president of ASCO, the organization of which Dr. Wright was a founding member, observed that "methotrexate forms the backbone of the first curative treatments for breast cancer and other cancers, as well as treatment for other serious diseases such as rheumatoid arthritis. And Jane did all this in the pre-modern era of molecular biology."

It was a Black woman who led the charge in advancing cancer treatment for all people at a time when the Civil Rights Act hadn't yet been passed. Her progress as a Black female physician-scientist began, even as the disastrous Tuskegee experiment was in full swing, in 1932. A Black woman who understood that new approaches were needed. She was not bothered by the fact that she was a Black female and a surgeon playing in a field dominated by White men. In fact, she's reported to have said those observations were of no concern to her. She was a healer, a scientist, and a clinical trialist in the driver's seat of oncology drug development that would one day be of great benefit to her people.

In 1971, the War on Cancer burst into the national consciousness. But what was the strategy? How would we win the fight? The National Cancer Institute, founded in 1937, would be the quarterback of the government's effort to push back against the invading force of cancer. With increased funding and direct access to the President of the United States, fifteen cancer centers across the country were authorized to develop cancer control programs and to plan, develop, and coordinate a national cancer strategy. Mary Lasker's dream was becoming a reality.

One remarkable and far-reaching result of this mandate was the founding of the Surveillance, Epidemiology, and End Result Program (SEER). SEER's directive was to monitor the burden of cancer: its trends, racial demographics, and survival rates. They also responded to public concerns and inquiries. SEER was for the people and was expected to respond to the needs of all the people—a huge mandate. It was no surprise that there was a rising cancer rate across all demographics. But it was becoming increasingly clear that there were sharp differences in both the incidence and mortality between Blacks and Whites. The incidence was higher for Blacks, and the mortality rate was worse.

According to the late Colin Powell, the first Black Joint Chief of Staff, before going to war, eight things should be considered. Among them:

- Is a vital national security interest threatened?
- Do the American people support the action?
- Do we have a clear, attainable objective?
- Have the risks and costs been fully and frankly analyzed?
- Have the consequences of our actions been fully considered?

As this relates to the War on Cancer, the answer to the first and second was yes. As for the last three, there was controversy from the beginning. There was an outcry against another government-funded endeavor. The naysayers opined, "The war is ill-fated, and such massive funding to the NCI would reduce funding to the other institutes of the NIH." They also said, "The definition of what constitutes victory isn't well defined." Some felt that the Laskers and others in their camp promoting this concept of a cancer campaign as "war" were out of their league. "What did they know about cancer, untrained as they were in the sciences?" Perhaps most concerning to some, they felt the whole strategy was foolhardy. Cancer isn't one disease, some correctly argued, so how can there be a war on "cancer"? To them, it made no sense. Just the mere thought of a "war" was misguided and simplistic. It may not be coincidental that this objection was made at a time when the increasingly unpopular war in Vietnam was raging.

As a side note, some of my hematology and oncology professors had been trained at and were, for a time, commissioned officers at the NCI before they joined the George Washington University faculty. I was fascinated by this and asked one of my more animated but brilliant mentors for some insight.

"Well, Fitzroy, many of us didn't want to go to Vietnam because we had strong objections to war in general and Vietnam in particular. We didn't want to be cannon fodder in a war that our government provoked. Many of us didn't have rich or well-connected relatives who could ensure we weren't drafted. Neither did we want to be carted off to jail as draft dodgers. This left us with two options. We could leave for Canada with the possibility of never returning home without facing jail time, or we could join the Commission Officer Corp of the NIH and fulfill our obligation of service. Some of us chose the latter."

The War on Cancer and the war of words raged on. Skirmishes were fought, and victories were won. And then suddenly, as if overnight, the decades-long research of Michael Bishop and Harold Varmus provided a quantum leap in our understanding of the very nature of what cancer is. The Nobel Prize in Physiology or Medicine 1989 was awarded jointly to J. Michael Bishop and Harold E. Varmus "for their discovery of the cellular origin of retroviral oncogenes."

The fundamental cause of cancer, they reasoned and subsequently demonstrated, results from normal cells in the body that go bad. Through their work, and subsequently that of others, we know that cancer arises from either autonomous expansion of either germline or somatic mutations of cells. In other words, germline mutations are cancer cell defects that are prone to cancer, which we inherit from our parent(s). These are already faulty cells, and they may become cancerous, no matter what we do to our bodies or what we are exposed to in the environment, such as the HER2/neu-gene. There may be other environmental factors that could accelerate the cancer process, but fundamentally, this is intrinsic to the cells some have inherited. The other, somatic mutation, is a direct result of environmental factors—carcinogens such as cigarette smoking, which leads normal lung cells to mutate due to chronic exposure to a series of toxic substances found in cigarettes.

Whether due to somatic or germline mutation, these flawed cells overcome the body's natural abilities to restrict cell growth. Mutated cells begin to take on a life of their own. They break down barriers and bend the human organs and systems to their will. The cells grow and multiply rapidly. They invade their neighbors and suppress and overwhelm the body's natural defenses to fight cancer, the immune system. Bizarrely, mutated cancer cells maintain many characteristics of normal cells but are altered enough to make them almost unrecognizable.

Unchecked cellular growth will retain some of the fundamentals of the tissue. Still, over time, their appearance and function become distorted and begin to inhibit and destroy the very organs in which they started.

Another way to look at this is to think of a family unit. Let's say a mom and dad have five children. They are taught the fundamentals of family values and the love of siblings, and they stand up and support each other. They are taught moral and religious values and respect for authority. The family members are similar in every way. That family minds its own business and doesn't interfere in the affairs of others. They're known and respected in their community.

FIGHTING FOR SURVIVAL

But, over time, there is one bad apple within that family. He goes astray, and the family exerts every effort to get him back on track, back to the fundamentals that have always marked the family. That son resists, and his behavior becomes increasingly bizarre and unpredictable. He's still a member of the family. His physical characteristics link him back to that specific family. But his behavior is increasingly erratic and unrecognizable. Ultimately, the family is ruined because that one son has had such a negative impact on them that they're no longer respected or recognized as an upstanding family in the community.

These distorted cells begin to multiply and dominate the other family of cells. Consequently, the family of cells is unable to carry out their original function. For instance, the lung's function is to exchange deoxygenated blood and replace it with oxygenated blood, something that's fundamental for human survival. With lung cancer, that function is increasingly compromised, and shortness of breath, bleeding, and coughing become early manifestations of lung cancer. The cancer's behavior is insatiable, and over time, it begins to negatively impact the whole neighborhood. Organs are overrun when these metastatic cells invade their neighbors, like the liver, brain, and bone. Over time, lung function worsens, and other body systems begin to fail. Unless effective treatment is found—surgery, chemotherapy, radiation therapy, or immunotherapy—the whole body falls apart, which results in death.

Bishop's and Varmus's revolutionary discovery was rocket fuel for cell biology and cancer research, and it dampened criticism of the War on Cancer for a while. Dr. Vincent DeVita, editor of our primary textbooks of oncology: *Cancer Principles and Practice of Oncology*—and for a time the director of the National Cancer Institute—had an upbeat impression of the war. He refuted the naysayers by saying, ". . . the 'War on Cancer' has had a profound impact and succeeded in fulfilling

153

its mandate. In the US, for example, overall incidence, mortality, and, in particular, morbidity from cancer have decreased, and relative survival rates for all cancers have increased 70 percent since the passage of the Act."

12

AUDACIOUS GOALS

*"That is America. Those bonds of affection; that common creed.
We don't fear the future; we shape it. We embrace it as one people,
stronger together than we are on our own."*

—President Barack Obama

I t's sobering to think that it's been fifty years since Nixon's
War on Cancer was brought to the national stage. That
said, billions of US taxpayer dollars have been spent, and
the rate of smoking among the young has decreased to a low
of 2.3 percent. More people are surviving a cancer diagnosis,
death rates from cancer have decreased by more than 30 percent, and early detection of lung cancer continues to improve.
Arguably, the NCI, charged with leading the national fight in
the early days, is an excellent source to learn how far we've
come. In 2021, on the fiftieth anniversary, the NCI listed
more than thirty substantial advances directly related to their

leadership and funding. These advances can be categorized under five major headings:

- A better understanding of the fundamentals of cancer cell formation
- Prevention and cancer risk reduction
- Personalized medicine beyond race
- Advances in immunotherapy
- Progress in breast cancer treatment

We will never be able to treat our way out of and put the country on a path to zero cancer by any timeline established by the federal government or any other agency, however laudable the goal is. Prevention, risk reduction, and early detection must be central to a zero-cancer strategy.

Many of my former patients and family members have often asked, and appropriately, "Why can't we prevent cancer? It's such a frightening disease." It's a relevant question that preoccupies health policymakers, primary physicians, insurers, and oncologists like me. I've heard this important question stated in a more pointed, cynical, and conspiratorial way by some: "You doctors and executives in the biotech industry know how to prevent and cure cancer, but you don't want to do it because you make more money from treating metastatic disease."

Of course, I can't entirely agree with this position, and I'm not aware of any conspiracy or collusion between physicians, scientists, and the drug industry. But I hear and understand the frustration. Indeed, the short answer is that many, but not all, cancers are preventable. Changes in personal lifestyles, such as the reduction in tobacco consumption, have led to a 25 percent reduction in tobacco-related mortality. But lung cancer death rates and late-stage presentation continue to be a significant factor in many Black communities. Many have argued that there's a direct relationship between advertising in some of these communities and the persistently high lung cancer rates. Obesity alone is responsible for 11 percent of all cancers. There's a large body of evidence that links obesity and the difficult-to-detect advanced cases of triple-negative breast cancer among Black women.

As a counter to the cynicism directed at the medical community, science-driven studies sponsored by the NCI have achieved significant results with respect to cancer risk reduction or prevention. Tamoxifen is a remarkable drug that was first approved for breast cancer treatment by the US FDA for years. Now, it plays a role in yet another milestone as we studied it as a breast cancer prevention agent in the Breast Cancer Prevention Trial (BCPT). At the end of this critical study, we were pleased to find that Howard University Cancer Center contributed the most significant number of African American study participants. This Phase 3 study was a potential game changer in *reducing the risk,* not *the treatment,* of breast cancer. The scientific question was: Could tamoxifen, a drug already approved for *the treatment* of breast cancer, also be effective in *reducing the risk of cancer?* The results from the study were an overwhelmingly positive "Yes!" Breast cancer risk could be reduced by almost 50 percent in women who took tamoxifen. This game-changing trial was not without controversy from the very beginning and is best summarized in 1995 by DeGregorio and others:

> The tamoxifen chemoprevention trial in healthy women is ongoing in over 250 cancer treatment centers. The use of tamoxifen for the treatment of postmenopausal women with known breast cancer has been touted as a medical breakthrough by many physicians. However, the ongoing trial, which enrolls high-risk healthy women above the age of 34, has been controversial since its initiation in 1991.

Congressional hearings, editorial, and statistical analyses concerning the scientific basis of the trial have emerged over the past year.

Taxpayer dollars funded this clinical trial. The US Congress authorized the funds used to conduct the trial. When complaints were made about the nature of the study and concerns were raised about the women's safety who were taking tamoxifen, they stepped in. There were hearings on Capitol Hill, and those responsible for the design and conduct of the trial had to answer questions. Happily, when the hearings were complete and the protocol was modified, the trial proceeded.

The BCPT study was followed by another breast cancer prevention trial called the STAR trial. The NCI also funded this clinical trial. The intent was to confirm or improve the BCPT results while using an even safer drug than tamoxifen. Instead of using a placebo, tamoxifen was compared to raloxifene. The STAR clinical trial showed that raloxifene was as effective as tamoxifen in reducing the risk of developing breast cancer. Just as important, raloxifene proved to be safer than tamoxifen. Because of this second study, post-menopausal women at risk for breast cancer had two FDA-approved drugs that could reduce the risk of breast cancer.

The topics of sex, sexually transmitted diseases, and cancer can make for difficult conversations, particularly among teens and preteens. The medical community knew there was a direct relationship between some sexually transmitted diseases and cancer of the cervix, vulva, penis, and anal cancer. All those cancers are associated with the human papillomavirus or HPV. According to the World Health Organization (WHO), there were over 600,000 cases of cervical cancer worldwide, which resulted in more than 300,000 deaths in 2020. Furthermore, WHO data points out that more than 90 percent of all cervical cancer is associated with HPV infection. Preventing infection or controlling it with a vaccine would be a significant victory for the United States and the world. Therefore, we had an excellent opportunity to reduce the risk and prevent cervical and other HPV-related cancers.

That knowledge led to an essential series of clinical trials that supported the clinical benefit of the HPV vaccine. As a result, the US FDA approved Gardasil, Ceravix*, and GARDISIL*9. All three drugs are administered as prophylaxis, or prevention, against HPV-related cancers. It's a fantastic achievement that required hundreds of participants over many years.

But with each advance comes controversy. The CDC recommends routine HPV vaccination as approved by the US FDA, starting at age nine. Some argued that discussing the vaccine with a child as young as nine would require conversations about sex. For many families, this is taboo.

"Why would I want to give my child a vaccine so young when I know they aren't having sex?" It's an uncomfortable subject for many, but others have said, "We don't care about these taboos. I must do all I can to protect my child before they go to high school or college." Unfortunately, clinical breakthroughs can be limited by a lack of societal acceptance.

In these last fifty years, cancer risk reduction and prevention have become considerable tools in the fight. Breast cancer and cervical cancer risk reduction are just two examples of how patient activism is shaping the future of cancer research. Colon and lung cancer reduction, brought about by early detection and treatment, are two more examples of how the fight against cancer is being fought and won.

"Caution: Cigarette Smoking May Be Hazardous to Your Health." This caution became law through yet another Act of Congress in 1965. Previously, some advertisers promoted the "medicinal benefits" of cigarettes. Still, despite the strong objection of the cigarette lobby, this new warning label was a significant step in warning the public about the dangers of tobacco products. Since then, the warnings have become more direct and blunt about the dangers. Now you'll see stronger warnings on every pack of cigarettes: "Smoking Causes Heart Disease, Emphysema . . . Cigarette Smoke Contains Carbon Monoxide." But we still have a long way to go. Lung cancer has the highest overall death rate of any cancer. The good news is that new cases of lung cancer have decreased because more people have quit smoking or never started.

For all those who continue to smoke or have quit, there's still a high risk of a first diagnosis. Through the efforts of NCI funding to scientists and clinician researchers, early detection through screening for lung cancer has come of age. As medical students, we received a twofold message: Counsel patients never to smoke, but if they do, tell them they should quit.

At first, a chest X-ray was the best tool we had to detect early-stage lung cancer. But it wasn't an effective method, and it was never supported by clinical research. Then, there was early data that suggested CAT scans might be a much more effective tool for finding early-stage lung cancer in heavy smokers. It was controversial at the time, but the NCI and other organizations funded multiple clinical trials that confirmed the early results. Nothing beats quitting or never smoking. But the next best thing is to find cancer in the early stage because, with surgery and other cancer treatments, many could be cured. In a 2020 *NEJM* article, de Koning and colleagues said, ". . . lung-cancer mortality was significantly lower among those who underwent volume CT screening than among those who underwent no screening at all."

Some years ago, Howard University Cancer Center and the hematology/oncology division of Howard University Hospital embarked on a colorectal screening program through community centers and churches. The pilot was intended to both educate the public about the benefits of cancer screening and to conduct a campaign. But screening for colon and prostate cancer involves, in part, an examination of the rectum with a gloved finger. Within these communities, digital rectal exams, proctoscopies, and colonoscopies are both a taboo for many, as well as a source of crass jokes about physicians who do these procedures. These are lifesaving procedures that many are too embarrassed to submit to.

I remember one presentation where the physician pointed out that "if blood is coming from your bum, run, do not walk to your primary physician ASAP." The physician knew this was a sign of colon cancer, and it was probably already very advanced. His statement was met with great laughter at the time. Even the thought of a self-administered, scientifically proven fecal-occult detection home kit wasn't well received. However, data shows that the lowly instrument reduces the incidence and death from colorectal cancer.

Patients, their advocates, government officials, and social policy professionals are quite correct in saying that more should be done to reduce cancer cases, even while we are advancing its treatment. All the above are great examples of how the War on Cancer is being won. We must continue to focus on public engagement and continued advocacy for prevention and other methods of cancer risk reduction.

In 1976, the great and dazzling American writer Tom Wolfe penned an essay titled "The 'Me' Decade and the Third Great Awakening." The essay chronicled the excesses, greed, and self-absorbance of the 1970s, which forever became known as the "Me Decade." Toward the end of the 1980s, as I was concluding my third and final year of a grueling internal medicine residency in Buffalo, New York, I had a rather casual but prescient

> We must continue to focus on public engagement and continued advocacy for prevention and other methods of cancer risk reduction.

conversation with a senior fellow. I told him that I'd won a hematology/oncology fellowship and that I was very excited and looked forward to taking a deeper dive into the subspecialties of hematology and oncology. He offered congratulatory remarks. That conversation morphed into the future of medical oncology as he understood it. Personalized medicine, he said, was the wave of the future, and medical oncology was the tip of the spear.

"Fitzroy," he said, "in the next ten years, the possibility of treating an individual based on his unique genetic and clinical profile is mind-blowing. Oncology is the future, despite how depressing and challenging it is to care for these patients now."

I appreciated his excitement, but at the time, I was interested in studying benign hematology. My interest in medical oncology then was more distant. Fast-forward more than thirty years since I first heard the term *personalized medicine,* and that concept has become fully baked into the fiber of the practice of medical oncology.

Sipuleucel-T, or PROVENGE° (US FDA approved in 2010 for prostate cancer), was a breakthrough that would lead to many other therapies fashioned for the individual patient. There are three basic but profound steps to deliver this treatment. First, cancer-fighting immune cells are removed from the patient diagnosed with prostate cancer. Second, those cancer-fighting immune cells are "turbo-charged" to make them even more powerful. Third, these more potent cells are returned to the original patient as a cancer-fighting vaccine.

The cells are tailor-made for that patient and no one else. If they are given to another individual with prostate cancer, it might not work and could lead to severe reactions. In that way, the cells are personalized. No two patients ever get the same vaccine; it's only effective for the patient from whom the immune cells were extracted.

Since then, five personalized anticancer agents that use a similar but different platform called CAR-T cell therapy have been approved by the US FDA with tongue-twisting names such as axicabtagene and tisagenlecleucel. CAR-T therapy leverages another type of cancer-fighting cells known as T-cells. They follow a similar path as PROVENGE*, where they're removed from the body, turbo-charged to make them more effective cancer-fighting warriors, and then returned to the individual cancer patient.

The PROVENGE* and the CAR-T platforms represent NCI-funded advances in personalized medicine and immunotherapy. But in 2011, the US FDA approved ipilimumab to manage metastatic melanoma. Until then, metastatic melanoma was almost always a death sentence. I knew of a Black physician and professor who was diagnosed with a rare form of melanoma in the early 2000s. Within months of the diagnosis, this brilliant physician was dead. Had he been diagnosed just ten years later, because of the advances in melanoma therapy, he might be alive today.

The approval of ipilimumab was a paradigm shift in the treatment of melanoma and a massive boost to the field of immunotherapy for cancers. Melanoma is an aggressive skin cancer that comes from excess sun exposure, especially in people originating in Northern Europe. The highest prevalence is in redheads or blonds who have green or blue eyes. Australians who are of Northern European descent have the highest rates of skin cancer overall. However, my story above shows that Black patients are also at risk. And the five-year survival rate was dismal.

I was the medical lead for a Phase 2 clinical trial to investigate a compound that targeted metastatic melanoma. At the time, many considered melanoma a graveyard diagnosis. The drug was ineffective for the treatment of melanoma, and our leadership decided to stop all research with the drug. Yet, there was some resistance among our team members because we felt that if we pushed a little harder, we could see some benefit.

Despite this failure, we knew that the prospects for metastatic melanoma were grim, and we desperately wanted to find a drug that would work. So, when the *NEJM* published the results of a definitive Phase 3 trial with ipilimumab, we sat up and took notice. A 20 percent five-year survival rate was reported, which meant that 20 percent of the patients studied were expected to be alive at five years. We couldn't believe it. Nothing that good had ever been reported before for metastatic melanoma.

To the nonparticipating investigator like me, the side effects of drug-induced diarrhea, pneumonitis, and nephritis—to name a few—were daunting. When I spoke to the participating investigators in Germany, I was told these were very manageable adverse events. I was still skeptical, but efficacy—measured by survival—was undeniable. Even for those who would later succumb to the disease, the radiologic improvements were eyepopping. These results led to the US FDA approval, which opened the way to even more incredible advances in the research and development of immune-oncology treatments for many cancers.

More than eight years ago, former US President Jimmy Carter was diagnosed with metastatic melanoma. In 2015, he received another type of immunotherapy, KEYTRUDA˚, and he's still alive as of this writing.

The diagnosis of metastatic melanoma is no longer a death sentence. I'm reminded of comments from the scientists and physicians who advised the US Senate as the War on Cancer legislation was being drafted. This comment stood out for me: "The long-term future may belong to the immunologist and the geneticist, the intermediate future to the chemotherapist, but the present and immediate future belong in the main to the surgeon and to some extent to the radiologist."

Immunology, perhaps the fourth arm of therapeutic oncology and hematology, has arrived and earned a seat at the table. The long-term future of immunotherapy has arrived. That future is now.

In 1975, the five-year breast cancer survival rate was 74 percent. In 2022, 90 percent of diagnosed women survive five years or more. Black women are not doing as well. Their five-year survival rate is 82 percent. Earlier breast cancer detection through self-examination and better screening methods, improved understanding of breast cancer biology, which drives better treatment options, and advances in breast cancer clinical trials have been major drivers contributing to the 16 percent increased survival rate. These improvements have been impressive, but more needs to be done.

Earlier, I mentioned that tamoxifen is an anti-estrogen, oral breast cancer therapy that kicked off a therapeutic revolution with its approval in 1978. It was first developed as a birth control agent, but after multiple clinical trials, it found a home as an effective therapy for post-menopausal women. Over the years of my practice, I've prescribed this drug to many post-menopausal women whose biopsied breast cancer tissue was positive for estrogen receptor (ER) or progesterone receptor (PR), which indicated they would respond very well to tamoxifen.

"Mrs. Jones, since your last visit and based on further analysis of your cancer, I have good news," I assured her.

"Believe me, Doctor, I need some good news," she said. "I've been worried that I may have to take chemo. My girlfriend had the same kind of breast cancer years ago, the same stage and everything, and her doctor told her she needed chemotherapy. I mean, I don't want chemotherapy. It's going to make my hair fall out. I'm going to be sick to my stomach, and I might need a blood transfusion and all that. But I'll do what I need to do to survive," she said.

"I have nice hair that came from my mother's side," she fretted. "Yeah, I know I'm vain, but I don't want to lose it."

"Well, no worries." I smiled. "Chemotherapy isn't necessary. All the studies say you should respond very well to tamoxifen if you stay on it for at least five years."

Still looking worried but less stressed, she broke in, "Come on, Doc, there must be side effects. I want to hear about that because I know that all drugs have side effects."

I explained to her that one of the most prominent problems women complain about is having hot flashes. Some complain about brain fog or chemo brain, which is associated with temporary memory loss, cloudy thought processes, and problems concentrating. Besides brain fog, I told her that tamoxifen could cause blood clots, and there was a low probability of cancer of the uterus that could first show up as vaginal bleeding. I assured her that since she'd already had a hysterectomy, she needn't be worried. I wrote a prescription, and she took the pills faithfully.

At around the five-year mark of Mrs. Jones's tamoxifen treatment, the NCI came out with a new recommendation based on new data that suggested that women who took tamoxifen for more than ten years showed improved survival. The recommendations also said that doctors should talk with their patients to discuss the pros and cons and then allow the patient to decide if they want to continue taking the medication. Remember, this was twice as long as I had recommended to Mrs. Jones five years before.

On a follow-up visit, I had a conversation with her. She wasn't happy. She wanted to be finished with the treatment and put her cancer in the rearview mirror. Taking a daily dose of anti-cancer medication reminded her every day of the thing she feared most. She wanted a second opinion.

"These are new recommendations," I told her. "Not every oncologist agrees with them, so if a second opinion would make you more comfortable, I encourage it."

I also referred her to the NCI website, where she could read and digest the information for herself. On a subsequent visit, she decided against further treatment. She was cancer-free, and she wanted to be done with treatment. However, she did agree to have regular checkup visits.

Government officials, the oncology community, scientists, patients, and cancer activists alike agree that the fight isn't over. But after the astonishing accomplishment of the last fifty years, many stalwarts of the field may even be crowing now, "So the war wasn't as wrongheaded as some had claimed."

They are partially correct. Those who lack resources, access to the best care, and limited health insurance have benefitted the least from these advances. Without question, understanding and targeting the biology of cancer has been a major step forward. But if it's out of reach for many, the battle for inclusion must continue.

With that in mind, in 2016, President Obama reignited the War on Cancer when he announced that then-Vice President Biden would ratchet up the fight. Mr. Biden had lost his oldest son, Beau Biden, to brain cancer in the prime of his life. The Vice President had a dog in the fight, and with that backdrop, Cancer Moonshot was launched. Like Obama's first campaign for the presidency in 2008, it was audacious in its scope: go faster to complete ten years' worth of work in only five. The nation could not and must not wait. Here are the goals:

1. All segments of society must have access to prevention strategies, diagnoses, and treatments that save lives.
2. Greater emphasis on converting incurable cancers into chronic diseases. The example for this goal was already set in the case of diabetes, which, before the discovery

of insulin by a Canadian researcher in 1920, was a death sentence.

3. Greater collaboration among physicians and scientists.
4. Healthcare professionals must see their patients as partners together.
5. Patients must have easy access to their health records.
6. Patients must have greater access to biomedical research and the use of their data.

It was overly ambitious in scope, perhaps, but the need was great. One of the signature departures from the past was the focus, not just on the science. In addition, patients must have a say in what will be done to their bodies and the tissues extracted. Do we think this was a dig at what happened at Tuskegee and at what happened to Mrs. Lacks? There's no question that these factors were on the mind of the Congress and their advisors. Patients and their advocates were empowered and authorized to ask questions—encouraged to seek the best care for themselves and their loved ones.

> Moonshot is an open invitation for patients to move off the sidelines and become participants in clinical care and clinical trials.

Obamacare was enacted before Moonshot, but clearly, having access to affordable care was part of the groundswell to be more inclusive. Moonshot is an open invitation for patients to move off the sidelines and become participants in clinical care and clinical trials.

Patients must resist their greatest fears, mistrust, and suspicions and begin to drive their role in the partnership with their physicians. Many more tools, unavailable in 1972, have been made available to make this possible.

CLAIM YOUR SEAT

"If they don't give you a seat at the table, bring a folding chair."

—Shirley Chisolm
(African American Presidential Candidate, 1972)

"You are young, gifted, and black. We must begin to tell
our young, 'There's a world waiting for you.
Yours is the quest that's just begun.'"

—Weldon Jonathan Irvine, Jr.

Dr. Valerie Montgomery Rice is an obstetrician/gyne-cologist and a highly respected researcher on women's health. She's also president and CEO of Morehouse School of Medicine in Atlanta, Georgia. In an online interview for *Washington Post Live*, "Exploring Health Equity: Clinical Trials," she responded to a question about low enrollment rates for African Americans and Latinos that "the messenger matters."

She went on to say why she had very high rates of enrollment of women while she was on faculty at the University of
Kansas:

> But that was because . . . I had a research coordinator who
> was African American, one who was Hispanic, and one who
> was Caucasian, and they went to the respective communi-
> ties, sometimes together, sometimes individually, to make
> sure that people saw someone who looked like them or that
> they could identify a relationship with. And that is how you
> build that trust.

Despite the significant lag in clinical trial enrollment rates
across the board, there have been some remarkable successes
and hope-elevating stories, which are fundamental to highlight,
even as there are sustained efforts to change the enrollment
trajectory.

US taxpayers fund the National Cancer Institute
Community Oncology Research Group (NCORP). In their
words, NCORP "is a national network of cancer care investigators, providers, academia, and other organizations that
provides care for diverse populations in healthcare systems."
Their emphasis is diversity and access within communities of
color, a very tangible manifestation of the federal government's
War on Cancer. While emphasizing access within communities of color, NCORP's leadership has partnered with academic
centers of excellence within these local communities. There are
local community sites in:

- Covington, Tennessee, with affiliated research sites in
  Arkansas and Mississippi
- New Orleans, Louisiana, with affiliate sites in Mississippi
- The Bronx, New York
- San Juan, Puerto Rico

This approach emphasizes a broad outreach to communities with significant health problems that have been ignored for years, respect for patients and their community leaders, and patient access to clinical trials that will make a difference in the lives of persons who have every reason to mistrust the system. I know from my years in academia that great ideas can die on the vine if there's not enough funding to get the research done. The approach has the full support and funding of the federal government to achieve success and to build trust within these disparate communities.

Patients have a right to be concerned that there should be greater attention given to conducting trials focused on preventing or reducing the risk of cancer. Referring to cancer metastasis, some patients have correctly pointed out that "once the horse is out the barn door, it's much harder to corral." Of course, patients have a personal responsibility in this regard, like quitting smoking, which will reduce the risk of lung cancer and cancer of the head and neck. It's also vital to good health to reduce obesity through better management of diet and exercise. A third approach over which patients have some control is to follow up with primary care physicians to ensure that universal guidelines regarding screening for colorectal, lung, breast, and prostate cancers get done.

NCORP is aligned with these concerns. NCORP, through the community-based initiatives described above, reports a 25 percent minority enrollment in all their funded clinical trials. This is a tremendous step forward compared to the national average of only 4 to 5 percent of eligible African Americans enrolling in cancer trials. With a five-time greater enrollment of minority patients, NCORP must be doing something right. These trials span the spectrum of cancer trials, from screening mammograms to new anti-cancer drugs.

Take, for example, the Tomosynthesis Mammographic Imaging Screening Trial (TMIST) study, a randomized breast cancer screening clinical trial that uses two different FDA-approved digital mammogram technologies. The goal is to determine which approach is better able to detect very early-stage breast cancer. And by the way, TMIST is an excellent example of a Phase 3 randomized trial that targets 130,000 women and seeks to answer an important question. It is significantly vital to Black women to know which type of mammogram is better for screening breast cancer because breast density impacts the ability of current screening procedures to successfully detect breast cancer. In April 2022, NCORP reported that 50 percent of the target was already screened, and an impressive 20 percent-plus were women of color.

The NCORP approach is positively impacting perceptions of clinical trials in Black communities. Conducting patient-ownership trials through community-based initiatives and making clinical trials available are all ways in which examples are being set. In addition, training the next generation of clinical trialists to serve their communities will further build trust and potentially change the low rates of current participation.

Many patients of color remain skeptical, and some are even hostile toward the biotech industry: "When I participate in a biotech-sponsored trial, what's in it for me?" For seventeen years, I've worked in research and development. My role in a team-wise approach is to identify hematologic and oncologic diseases in need of new drugs, develop ethical plans to study these drugs for the cancers identified, and conduct clinical studies that will determine if the drug works. We in the industry need to be more transparent and more intentional in winning the trust of many African Americans in particular. We also need to demonstrate in real terms that we have a shared interest in our communities

> The NCORP approach is positively impacting perceptions of clinical trials in Black communities.

and that this is not just a business. The industry needs to present itself as a long-term and sustained partner in the health and well-being of the community from which patients are recruited and clinical data is obtained, leading to drug approval. It must be viewed as ethical and socially committed "investors" in the community to obtain and sustain the trust.

But I have seen remarkable changes. When I entered the industry from my position at Howard University, one of the first challenges I wanted to consider was developing new drugs for sickle cell disease. At the time, hydroxyurea was the only US FDA-approved drug for patients diagnosed with sickle cell disease. There was no interest in developing anything new, but I continued to raise the question because I witnessed the severely painful crisis in some of the patients we cared for.

In rapid succession, within the last seven years, four additional drugs have been approved to treat sickle cell disease. Multiple biotech companies are pursuing better and less toxic agents. Gene therapy and bone marrow transplant or stem cell transplant with the possibility of cure are additional options for some patients. The progress in sickle cell research has not all been altruistic, but there are voices within the industry who are willing to ask hard questions and take substantial financial risks to answer them. In her interview with Frances Stead Sellers of the *Washington Post*, Dr. Rice expanded her comments by speaking to the pharma industry:

> I think the important thing is that we have to make sure that pharmaceutical companies understand that if we really want people to reach their optimal level of health, and we are going to have interventions like drugs or technology, we need to account for those differences that may occur when people are taking the drugs or utilizing the technology. And the only way you will know that is if you have the persons, those different people, participating in the clinical trials.

The US FDA has issued guidance for the industry for decades regarding the importance of diversity in clinical trials. The Open Public Hearing is often conducted by the US FDA prior to drug approval. This is where "Interested persons may present data, information, or views, orally or in writing, on issues pending before the committee."

I've attended some of these meetings, both in person and online, when new drugs are reviewed. On one occasion, a new drug application for ovarian cancer was under review by the US FDA. The results of the study were very positive, and more women benefitted from the new drug in comparison to the standard treatment. In the public hearing segment, one woman stood up, gathered herself, stepped to the microphone, and launched into a tirade. She was passionate in her objection to the approval of the new drug. She agreed with the positive findings of the study. She did not seem to have any objections about the safety profile of the drug. She railed against approval because the population studied was not diverse, and most of the women, as is often the case with many industry-led trials, were White. She said since the study participants did not represent the racial and ethnic diversity of the United States, its actual benefit to all women with ovarian cancer was not established. On the strength of that argument, she opposed approval. Incidentally, the woman was White.

At that point, the US FDA had multiple options. First, they could approve the drug, which, happily, they did. Second, they could limit approval to White women since they were the largest group studied. A third option was to reject approval altogether, which was the preferred option for the speaker at the microphone. A fourth option that wasn't presented at the time was to insist that the company applying for drug approval conduct a post-approval study with a more diverse participant pool to evaluate the safety and efficacy results and then submit it to the FDA for review. This second study could provide evidence that the drug was either equally effective for these groups or not. The problem with the speaker's preference, although well intended, was that it could potentially deny benefits to some Black women when there was no scientific basis to believe Black women wouldn't benefit. To her point, if approved, doctors could be prescribing a drug to people of color without any data that supported it had a positive effect or could reduce harm.

The industry has been under increasing pressure to address these concerns. Speaking again from my experience, some biotech companies allocate meaningful sums of their study budget to ensure a better enrollment outcome for African Americans and other people of color, with mixed results. Others seem to be going through the "check the box" motions only.

Besides proclamations about the importance of clinical trial diversity, the US FDA has gone even further. In 2020, the FDA (the Agency) published "Enhancing the Diversity of Clinical Trial Populations—Eligibility Criteria, Enrollment Practices, and Trial Designs Guidance for Industry." In it, the Agency doubled down on its desire to see clinical trials done in the United States "better reflect the population most likely to use the drug if the drug is approved." The guide states that the demographic of race, sex, age, and geographic location of participants in clinical trials should be captured. Of equal importance, the Agency asks sponsors to consider and include participants at the "extremes of the weight range," persons with disabilities, and persons who were diagnosed with AIDS but were otherwise medically stable and functioning well despite their diagnosis. Many of the recommendations are common sense and, if followed, would increase patient diversity. Sponsors want a drug that has great clinical benefits with minimal side effects and one that will increase the possibility that the Agency will approve it. On the other hand, a population too narrowly defined from a regulatory agency point of view may not give a clear indication of its actual effect on the broader population if approved.

Years ago, a company I worked for conducted a Phase 1 clinical trial in patients diagnosed with sickle cell disease. We excluded patients who were known to be HIV positive because the medication frequently used could cause severe side effects if taken with the research drug. On the other hand, if excluding such patients is routine, we may never know if a newly approved drug will help those patients.

The COVID-19 pandemic and the murder of George Floyd in 2020 were seismic events that touched every aspect of our society, including the biotech industry. In November 2020, nine months after WHO declared COVID-19 a pandemic and just six months after Floyd's death, the pharmaceutical industry issued the "first-ever, industry-wide principles on clinical trial diversity." The stated goals were:

- Building trust and acknowledging the historic mistrust of clinical trials within Black and Brown communities.
- Reducing barriers to clinical trial access.
- Using real-world data to enhance information on diverse populations beyond product approval.
- Enhancing information about diversity and inclusion in clinical trial participation.

By April 2021, the proposal was approved, which was lightning speed for a conservative organization perceived to be primarily driven by a profit motive. What drove this apparent about-face? The people I've spoken to felt this was nothing short of a public relations campaign. For years, the industry withstood withering criticism from the public, public interest groups, physicians, and government agencies. Others believe that this was a genuine about-face that reflected that the industry now recognizes and embraces that they do have societal responsibility. It fits into the rising demand for social justice.

We know that besides national leaders such as Dr. Anthony Fauci, leaders from the industry C-Suite were making major pitches to African American communities to participate in COVID-19 trials. One practical outcome was a $10 million grant intended as initial support for an eighteen-month pilot in ten sites across the US. The sites were Morehouse School of Medicine, Yale School of Medicine, Vanderbilt University Medical Center, and the Research Centers in Minority Institutions Coordinating Center at Morehouse School of Medicine.

"Our goal," said Ramona Sequeira, Chair of PhRMA board of directors, "is to make sure all people, regardless of geography, socioeconomics, race, ethnicity or gender identity, who want to participate in a clinical trial have the opportunity to do so."

About a year ago, I spoke to a Meharry faculty member and a former Howard University colleague who knew about the Vanderbilt initiative. He spoke highly of the program, the potential impact on Black patients in the Nashville area, and the possibility of a shot in the arm for clinical research.

Since then, there's been increasing activity, grants, funding, and speeches by leading pharmaceutical companies that followed the lead of the industry. Pfizer Pharmaceutical, in collaboration with Columbia University in New York City, funded the Columbia-Pfizer Clinical Trials Diversity Initiative. They gave a $10 million grant with the stated goal of improving diversity in clinical trial participants. Rod Mackenzie, Executive Vice President and Chief Development Officer at Pfizer, said, "Diversity of representation in clinical trials is a matter of equity, which is a core Pfizer value. We are deeply committed to ensuring our clinical trials reflect the diversity of the communities like New York in which they are conducted." A primary concern raised by those who've studied and lived with these challenges is that there's this burst of interest and a stated commitment to clinical study diversity participation. One longtime leader in the field sounded a cautionary note. To paraphrase him, he said we need to be careful not to assume that these grants will be a magic wand for clinical study diversity. It isn't like we'll snap our fingers, and there will be a ready pool of minority patients to draw from or ready access to patients to meet a predefined diversity quota. It will require well-designed strategies and execution.

Will this support from the industry be sustained if these expectations are not met? Minority communities will be paying attention because, again, there's a concern that the industry has a short attention span and hasn't always shown a sustained interest in their communities.

The African American participation in clinical trials, generally agreed to be about 4 percent, has not changed in the last thirty or more years. In 2021, Serena Tharakan, a medical student at the Icahn School of Medicine, published a paper in the journal *Cancer*: "The impact of globalization of cancer clinical trials on the enrollment of Black patients." Independently, they confirmed the traditionally low rates of enrollment. Did higher rates of patient enrollment outside the United States have an impact on the low enrollment of Black participants in the US? Their study attempted to provide an answer. They reported that between 2015 and 2018, forty-nine cancer drugs were approved by US FDA. There was a significant decrease in African American enrollment, which the authors believe was due to globalization, in that it's often easier and more efficient to recruit patients outside the United States who cross all races. Tharakan and colleagues concluded that clinical trials conducted primarily outside the United States were much less likely to enroll Black patients compared to trials conducted in the United States. Consequently, she and others suggest that the true safety and efficacy of these approved drugs may not be known in an African American context. This suggests that the industry must redouble the effort to enroll more African Americans as well as other Americans.

The biotech industry is a business that's subject to some of the same challenges as any other business: time, competition, creating a product, and being first to market. Michael Rosenblatt, a physician and former CEO of a large pharmaceutical company, provides a perspective on the complexities and challenges the industry faces in getting a drug approved by regulatory bodies such as the US FDA. In a 2017 *NEJM* article titled "The Large Pharmaceutical Perspective," he writes:

> **The African American participation in clinical trials, generally agreed to be about 4 percent, has not changed in the last thirty or more years.**

Large pharmaceutical companies conduct clinical trials to evaluate efficacy and identify safety issues for candidate drugs as effectively, efficiently, and expeditiously as possible while addressing simultaneously the requirements of regulatory authorities across the globe. To put the fewest people at risk and to learn the most, these trials often are configured to provide evidence for health care providers, regulatory approval, and reimbursement from health agencies. Because there are so many unknowns, pharmaceutical research and development is a high-risk business with the highest failure rate for new product candidates in any industry.

This could very well be viewed as a self-serving statement. And I'm not sure that most patients want to hear all the details of what goes on in the inner recesses of the industry's decision-making. However, Rosenblatt says there are many "masters" that need to be served on the path to a successful drug launch, each of which has their unique demand, and satisfying the regulatory body is one of the most significant masters. Demands for greater diversity are only one of many.

Investing $19 million in a single failed cancer trial may not break the bank of a large drug company. On the other hand, many of the innovations driving biotech today come from small companies. A 10 percent success rate for oncology drugs meeting regulatory standards is a 90 percent failure rate that can and has broken the backs of some smaller companies. Dr. Richard Mosicki and colleagues capture that sentiment in another *NEJM* article from February 2017. They observe:

> Small biopharmaceutical companies often encounter important challenges in designing and implementing clinical development programs. In a context in which only approximately 10 percent of clinical programs result in drugs that achieve regulatory approval, small-company clinical programs may have an even lower rate of success than that of large companies owing to limited internal experience in clinical development and limited infrastructure, which may also affect manufacturing and clinical supply.

These points aren't frequently discussed in public spaces because, in a sense, it's the cost of doing business. But to drive future innovation and risk-taking, having this dialogue is in the interest of the nation's health. The industry needs to lift the veil if they are to continue to build trust. Patients need to lean in and peer behind the veil to better understand the complexities of the industry. Some companies invite the public to take a seat at the decision-making table so they'll understand some of the issues, raise objections, and be better positioned to understand the tremendous value of the industry. Others will need to pull up a chair, take a seat at the table, and invite themselves.

African American patients want to see that clinical trials aren't only about the bottom line. The messenger, the message, and the messaging matter.

Some have criticized the industry because the C-Suite doesn't seem to have enough seats at the table to accommodate people who can give greater insights into the diversity question. Recently, Larry Fink, Founder, Chairman, and CEO of BlackRock, published a letter calling for greater social responsibility among American Corporations. Quoting from his 2018 Letter to CEOs, he says, "Companies must benefit all of their stakeholders, including shareholders, employees, customers, and the communities in which they operate." Concerning corporate board diversity, he stressed, "We also will continue to emphasize the importance of a diverse board. Boards with a diverse mix of genders, ethnicities, career experiences, and ways of thinking have, as a result, a more diverse and aware mindset." This is a considerable shortcoming among corporations focused on health. The health concerns and health disparities that are so glaring and so obvious to some may not

But there's another actor in all of this. It's the Black patient who's diagnosed with cancer. They must also respond in their best interest.

be visible to board members because of sheer ignorance.

Putting aside cynicism, I believe strides are being made. If this push by the industry is sustained and accelerated, the profile of the patients recruited could change dramatically over the next five to ten years. Unfortunately, we are not there yet.

But there's another actor in all of this. It's the Black patient who's diagnosed with cancer. They must also respond in their best interest. There's no question that many have been and continue to be victimized by the original sin of slavery that's still with us. Pivoting away from the past, rejecting fear and mistrust, and finding a path when there sometimes seems to be none is also our burden. The fear of missing out on the medical revolution taking place must be a driver. For themselves, their children, and future generations, change must begin within the community. There are heroes among you. Taking a page from Maya Angelou's brilliant book, *I Know Why the Caged Bird Sings*, "The need for change bulldozed a road down the center of my mind."

14

HOPE IS ALIVE

*"Often, when people hear the word cancer or leukemia, they are
scared, both because they don't know a lot about the disease,
and they don't know what is going to happen to them.
Some immediately think it's a death sentence.
I know these feelings first-hand because that's what I thought."*

—Kareem Abdul Jabbar

The last forty years of healthcare in the US have been
turbulent, exhilarating, and groundbreaking. For
example, the cancer death rate since 1991 has decreased
by 33 percent. As of 2022, in the United States, more than 18
million persons are cancer survivors. A closer look is even more
astonishing: 67 percent of all cancer survivors are over the age
of sixty-five, and 47 percent of all cancer survivors have lived
more than ten years since their initial diagnosis. Has the War
on Cancer, kicked off by an ACT of Congress in 1972, been

won? The emphatic answer is no. There is so much more to do, but these statistics suggest progress is being made.

As impressive as the improved cancer data are, these last four decades have been book-ended by two terrifying global health events that seemed to come out of nowhere with the overwhelming power of a tsunami that swept many to their death. First, the dawn of the 1980s overwhelmed the world with the AIDS epidemic and the death and destruction it brought. The second was the COVID-19 pandemic, which enveloped the globe at the dawn of the 2020s. Nations were incarcerated in economic lockdown, finger-pointing, and panic. Both cataclysmic events triggered never-ending conspiracy theories based on misunderstandings, half-truths, and mistrust of national governments. COVID-19 rumors were turbocharged by universal access to the internet. Yet, through it all, brilliant physicians, clinical trialists, scientists, and altruistic patients made extraordinary sacrifices to advance clinical medicine in the interest of the greater good. They led the way from an initial response of despair through the unknown swamp of never-before-described diseases to a brighter day for people living with AIDS and those diagnosed with COVID-19.

The AIDS crisis, horrific both in scope and the savagery with which it consumed its victims, will forever be linked to the heroic efforts of medical and scientific giants. Giants such as Anthony Fauci, head of the National Institutes of Allergy and Infectious Diseases, was a lynchpin in the federal government's early strategy against AIDS. Brilliant scientists such as Luc Montagnier, a Frenchman, were credited with co-discovering HIV, for which he was the co-Nobel Laureate awarded in 2008.

However, we must remember the heroic patients who did not succumb, nor did they give in without a fight. On the patient side, the fight against AIDS had no more prominent name than Irving "Magic" Johnson, the Basketball Hall of

Famer and LA Lakers multiple-NBA championship winner. Arguably the American poster child, he showcased how far AIDS research and treatment has progressed since the painfully unforgettable 1980s. According to Steven Taranto of CBSSports.com, Magic "has become a living testament to advances in medicine that have turned human immunodeficiency virus (HIV) from a death sentence into something that can be managed and lived with. While Johnson can now attest to 30 years of life after being diagnosed with HIV, his journey living with the disease has been far from easy."

Furthermore, when Magic Johnson commented on his decision to play on the gold-winning 1992 US Olympic Men's Basketball Dream Team (after he was diagnosed with AIDS), he said, "It proved to be the right decision. . . It helped people who were living with not just HIV and AIDS, but with any other disease, that you can live on; you can live a productive life."

And what a productive life he's had! After his playing days were over, he continued to surge. He was at different times the head coach of the LA Lakers, president of the LA Lakers Basketball Operations, and part owner of the LA Dodgers, the winners of the 2020 Baseball World Series. He was also a United Nations Ambassador of Peace.

When I started my tenure at Howard University, I'd already completed three years as a hematology/oncology fellow who observed, diagnosed, and treated primarily young men diagnosed with two AIDS-related cancers: non-Hodgkin lymphoma (NHL) and Kaposi's sarcoma. I made it known that I was very comfortable managing these cancer challenges based on my prior experience and the limited therapeutic tools available at the time.

As a result, a significant number of Black men diagnosed with AIDS-related cancers and admitted to our hospital in the early 1990s were referred to my clinical practice. But to successfully manage these diseases meant that there had to be a dramatic improvement in their weakened immune system caused by the virus. Yet, my team and I soldiered on with the best treatment options available, none of which had meaningful long-term benefits for these AIDS-related cancers.

Very little was published regarding how to treat patients, and what little there was, was of limited benefit. But over five years—it seemed like it happened overnight—the number of patients in my practice dwindled from a steady flow to a trickle—and finally to none at all. When the trend became clear, my reaction was to seek answers that explained the dramatic decline. I considered the following possibilities: Maybe patients and referring physicians lost confidence in my abilities as an oncologist. Or perhaps patients were spontaneously getting better. The answers to those questions and many others that churned through my mind were put to rest by the facts.

The facts were that by the mid-1990s, a substantial reason for the dramatic decline was the introduction of highly active antiretroviral therapy, or HAART, made available between 1995 and 1996. The CDC reports: "From 1981 through 1990, 100,777 deaths among persons with acquired immunodeficiency syndrome (AIDS) were reported to by local, state, and territorial health departments; almost one-third (31,196) of these deaths were reported during 1990." With the introduction of HAAT in 1996, the annual AIDS death rate decreased by 78 percent.

This HAART cocktail of highly effective agents that battled against the AIDS virus improved the human immune system of infected patients. With an improved immune system, the body's natural defenses against infections and cancer were restored. Now, with a liberated immune system, the body was poised to fight back against Kaposi's sarcoma and non-Hodgkin lymphoma, thus rendering chemotherapies unnecessary. The breakthrough success didn't occur by random happenstance. Instead, it came about through hard-nosed scientific experiments, patient advocacy groups, and the US FDA's willingness to revisit and accelerate their processes for approving new drugs.

Regarding patient advocacy, Peter Staley, a self-described political activist and an early member of the AIDS Coalition to Unleash Power (ACT UP), wrote an opinion piece for the *New York Times* in December 2022. In it, he outlines the multiple conversations and conferences he and members of ACT UP had with Dr. Anthony Fauci, hoping to advance AIDS research and access to potentially effective AIDS medications that were still in development but not yet approved by the US FDA. In the opinion piece and with homage to Dr. Fauci, he says:

> Days after the conference, I found myself in Dr. Fauci's office, along with the ACT UP members Mark Harrington and Jim Eigo, hammering out the final details of our parallel track program, which would allow thousands of people to obtain experimental drugs outside of traditional clinical trials. Within days, a *New York Times* front page headline about Dr. Fauci read, "AIDS Researcher Seeks Wide Access to Drugs in Tests." The F.D.A. (sic) quickly fell in line. ACT UP had scored its first major victory . . .

The willingness of patients, both Blacks and Whites, to stare down death itself, make decisions that they wanted to live, and participate in clinical trials was a powerful way to advocate for themselves. The effect has been nothing short of astounding for the various AIDS communities. In fact, the changes made in the drug approval process, based on ACT UP and other advocacy groups, have had positive long-term consequences on cancer drug development in the US.

While it remains a problem, HIV infection is no longer the major health scare it used to be. Effective treatment is available. Americans across all ethnicities, races, and political and religious persuasions have banded together to fight against and battle the twin scourges of HIV and COVID-19.

Black Americans and their leaders are raising their voices to advocate for more resources and more access to clinical trials—clinical trials that matter to them and that are perceived to be in their best interest. Data from the NCORP clinical trials is clear evidence that Black Americans will participate in clinical trials when investigators are committed to their interests and communities. They will participate when the barriers of mistrust and disrespect are broken down. Many Black Americans understand the importance of paying it forward through clinical trials. Many have said as much.

> Black Americans and their leaders are raising their voices to advocate for more resources and more access to clinical trials—clinical trials that matter to them and that are perceived to be in their best interest.

Just like the War on Cancer launched in 1971, there's more financial support for clinical trials for poor and underserved communities who want to participate in clinical trials. We now know more about the unique features of prostate cancer and breast cancer, as well as multiple myeloma in Black communities. This is hope—hope based on scientific data and the volunteerism of African Americans willing to participate in finding answers to their cancer problems.

The 1971 Act of Congress that spawned the War on Cancer gave rise to the Surveillance, Epidemiology, and End Results (SEER) Program, which was charged with the study, documentation, and reporting of cancer statistics for all Americans. Part of that charge is to compare ethnic, racial, and geographic trends over time. SEER data over the decades has consistently documented differences in cancer trends, indicating there are continued significant cancer disparities by race and ethnicity.

What sometimes gets lost in the discussion are the positive steps African Americans take year after year, despite the odds, to help themselves. Between 1993 and 2019, Black versus White disparities in mortality rates in colorectal, prostate, breast, and other cancers have been narrowed with an overall downward

> This is hope—hope based on scientific data and the volunteerism of African Americans willing to participate in finding answers to their cancer problems.

trend. Consistent with these trends and to the credit of African Americans, we also see remarkable steps forward in that HPV vaccination to prevent or reduce the risk of the multiple cancers mentioned in Chapter 11 is essentially no different compared to Whites. The rates of cervical cancer, breast cancer, and colorectal cancer screening are also very comparable. African Americans should celebrate the efforts they have made in these areas.

But of course, there's more work to be done toward improved cancer risk reduction, which should be the first order of business. We must reject the fear of cancer and embrace the impressive treatment options currently available. And finally, we must accept that some clinical answers to the cancers that plague African Americans will only come when we embrace the potential benefits of cancer research in all its forms.

I once took care of a diplomat from West Africa, a man in his early forties with a young family who was diagnosed with acute promyelocytic leukemia (APL). APL was once considered one of the most aggressive leukemias with a dismal prognosis. He was treated with the anti-leukemic drug All-Trans Retinoic Acid (ATRA), the standard of care at the time. All cancer medications, including ATRA, have side effects, and some patients experience a unique syndrome called APL syndrome that includes fever, shortness of breath, massive weight gain, lung infiltrates, and cardiac issues. If not quickly recognized, it could lead to death. He was treated with high doses of steroids, recovered, and was discharged from the ICU. The last time I saw him, he was doing well. He was cured of leukemia and looked forward to returning home to West Africa. From the early days when APL was first described, to the 1980s when ATRA was first used by the Chinese, to the present day, the cure rate for APL is now greater than 90 percent.

Yes, hope is alive. And as long as African Americans take their hard fought and well-deserved seat at the table and participate in proven cancer prevention measures—and clinical trials—we can expect to enjoy the benefits and be instrumental in the fight to conquer cancer.

ACKNOWLEDGMENTS

L et me say at the very outset that I owe an extraordinary debt of gratitude to all African Americans, particularly those brave souls who have suffered and are suffering from cancer. They have challenged and inspired me to become a better medical oncologist and clinical trialist. They inspired this book, and it is with great appreciation that by allowing me to walk alongside them, I was moved to write this book. This book is my love letter to them.

Next, I want to thank my African American wife, who helped me, a Jamaican-born Black man, understand the complexities of what it means to be African American with all the diversity, highs and lows, tremendous challenges, and triumphant joys! Her steady, unwavering support and encouragement have been infectious.

This book would not be possible without the many professors and researchers who have inspired me over more than thirty years. To these, I owe my gratitude: the late Dr. Gerald L. Logue, Professor of Medicine in the Division of Hematology, Jacobs School of Medicine and Biomedical Sciences, Buffalo, New York; Professor Geraldine Schechter; the late Lawrence Lessin, MD of George Washington University School of Medicine, who taught me how to approach the art and science of medicine with compassion and rigor; and Professor James Ahlgren, rocket scientist turned medical oncologist, who was the primary clinical investigator I most wished to become when I was a young hematology/oncology fellow.

I can't say enough about my mentor and good friend, Professor Victor Gordeuk of the University of Illinois, Chicago, a hematologist extraordinaire. He taught me to write scientifically. When I asked, "How many drafts does one need before submitting a research paper?" he responded, "As many as it takes." He taught me to hold my own in any rigorous scientific or medical debate and to challenge dogma with data.

I've written many medical abstracts and clinical science papers. Writing a book to educate and inspire is another matter entirely. In my writing coach and editor, Nancy Erickson, I found a thoughtful and patient teacher who would never let a good book die. She said I had a book in me. I began to believe it, and she helped me to find it. Nancy—thank you.

ABOUT THE AUTHOR

Fitzroy Dawkins, MD, is a medical oncologist and hematologist with over thirty years of experience as a practitioner, teacher, clinical researcher, and biotech tech executive. He completed a three-year fellowship in hematology and medical oncology at George Washington University Medical Center in Washington, DC. He began his career as an Assistant Professor of Medicine at Howard University College of Medicine, with the appointment as attending physician in hematology and medical oncology at Howard University Hospital.

When AIDS-related Kaposi sarcoma and non-Hodgkin lymphoma were rampant in the African American community, he was there. When the scourge diminished due to advanced clinical research, he was there. For fourteen years, he was relentless in making the case that African Americans diagnosed with cancer must begin to heal themselves by confronting the risks associated with cancer, aggressively pursuing the best cancer care possible, and embracing clinical trials. He also saw the hope, courage, and resilience of many African Americans who took charge of their health and were willing to engage in the fight to save their lives.

Dr. Dawkins is the author of multiple papers and abstracts in the *New England Journal of Medicine*, *Journal of Clinical Oncology*, and the medical journal *Blood*, among others.

For the past eighteen years, he's worked as an executive with increasing roles and responsibilities at Johnson & Johnson in Medical Affairs and R&D, Incyte Corporation, and most recently as Vice President of Clinical Development at Forma Therapeutics in Watertown, Massachusetts. In the biotech industry, Dr. Dawkins has tirelessly advocated for more funding and increased sensitivity in clinical research recruiting and retention methods across all disease types, from Black patients diagnosed with pancreatic cancer to those with inherited sickle cell disease. He's helping the industry understand that the mistrust that African Americans have is deep and well founded and that the industry must win their trust if recruiting efforts are to succeed.

His book is intended to change the mindset of African Americans from mistrust to participation in the phenomenally positive revolution that is taking place in biomedical sciences and clinical research. He makes the case that many of the healthcare issues facing African Americans can be solved through research, but they must aggressively demand a place at the table. African Americans must begin to heal themselves against all odds.

Currently, Dr. Dawkins is a principal medical consultant with Data Revive, USA, LLC. He lives in the Princeton, New Jersey, area with his wife of over thirty years. He has two daughters who have successfully launched their careers in the tech industry.